P9-DUD-788

CONTENTS

Eating Well with
Diabetes

By Mary Jane Finsand,
Edith White, M.Ed.,
Karin Cadwell, Ph.D., R.N.

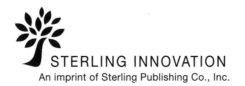

STERLING INNOVATION
An imprint of Sterling Publishing Co., Inc.

New York / London
www.sterlingpublishing.com

STERLING, the Sterling Logo, STERLING INNOVATION,
and the Sterling Innovation logo are registered trademarks
of Sterling Publishing Co., Inc.

Library of Congress Cataloging-in-Publication Data Available

2 4 6 8 10 9 7 5 3 1

Published by Sterling Publishing Co., Inc.
387 Park Avenue South, New York, NY 10016

© 2010 by Sterling Publishing Co., Inc.

This book is comprised of material from the following Sterling titles:
The Complete Diabetic Cookbook © 1987 by Sterling Publishing Co., Inc.
Great Diabetic Desserts & Sweets © 1995 by Karin Cadwell and Edith White
Diabetic Candy, Cookie & Dessert Cookbook © 1982 by Mary Jane Finsand

Distributed in Canada by Sterling Publishing
c/o Canadian Manda Group, 165 Dufferin Street
Toronto, Ontario, Canada M6K 3H6
Distributed in the United Kingdom by GMC Distribution Services
Castle Place, 166 High Street, Lewes, East Sussex, England BN7 1XU
Distributed in Australia by Capricorn Link (Australia) Pty. Ltd.
P.O. Box 704, Windsor, NSW 2756, Australia

Printed in China
All rights reserved

Sterling ISBN 978-1-4027-7341-9

For information about custom editions, special sales, premium and
corporate purchases, please contact Sterling Special Sales
Department at 800-805-5489 or specialsales@sterlingpublishing.com.

INTRODUCTION

Eating Well with Diabetes was created to help beginning as well as more experienced cooks by adding to their repertoire of diabetic recipes. No one wants to think of him or herself as being on a restricted diet, yet all of us are on a diet; therefore, it is the word "restricted" which must be removed. This cookbook is designed to remove the word "restricted," to give a more tasteful and varied food intake for everyone. It is meant to reduce and simplify the day-to-day preparation of healthful, good food. There are no complete menus, but rather individual recipes that will open up new cooking horizons. By using the simple EXCHANGE or caloric values, anyone can whip up a gourmet meal with no fear of overindulgence.

If you look at the number of savory and sweet recipes, you will notice that the dessert section is nearly as large as the rest of the book. This reflects the fact that there are so many people with a sweet tooth, and many more who do not feel a meal is complete without dessert.

Eating a piece of pie or a candy bar without knowing the EXCHANGE value or calorie count can be disastrous to any diet. All of us should be aware of our total calorie intake and compare it to our total calorie output daily. To make weight reduction or a healthy diet as pleasant as possible, it is important to realize that eating can still be made an enjoyable experience.

It would be an overstatement to suggest that this cookbook has all the answers to feeding a diabetic. It does not. However, *Eating Well with Diabetes* will help family cooks form everyday good eating habits for the diabetic and for the rest of the family as well.

Using the Recipes for Your Diet

All recipes have been developed using diet substitutions for sugar, syrup, sauces, toppings, puddings, gelatins, mayonnaise, salad dressings, and imitation or lo-cal dairy and non-dairy products.

Remember, diet is the key word for controlling diabetes, and each person's diet is prescribed individually by a doctor or counselor who has been trained to mold your daily life to your diet requirements. DO NOT try to outguess them. If you have any questions about any diabetic recipes, ask your diet counselor.

Read the recipes carefully, then assemble all equipment and ingredients. "Added Touch" ingredients are flavorful additions, but not necessary to the recipe's success. Substitutions or additions of herbs and spices or flavorings to a recipe may be made by using the guide for Spices and Herbs, or for Flavorings and Extracts; they will make any of the recipes distinctively your own.

Use standard measuring equipment (whether metric or customary), and be sure to measure accurately. Remember, these recipes are good for everyone, not just the diabetic.

CUSTOMARY TERMS		METRIC SYMBOLS	
t.	teaspoon	mL	milliliter
T.	tablespoon	L	liter
c.	cup	g	gram
pkg.	package	kg	kilogram
pt.	pint	mm	millimeter
qt.	quart	cm	centimeter
oz.	ounce	C	Celsius
lb.	pound		
F	Fahrenheit		
in.	inch		

GUIDE TO APPROXIMATE EQUIVALENTS

Customary: Metric:

ounces; pounds	cups	tablespoons	teaspoons	milliliters	grams; kilograms
			¼ t.	1 mL	
			½ t.	2 mL	
			1 t.	5 mL	
			2 t.	10 mL	
½ oz.		1 T.	3 t.	15 mL	15 g
1 oz.		2 T.	6 t.	30 mL	30 g
2 oz.	¼ c.	4 T.	12 t.	60 mL	
4 oz.	½ c.	8 T.	24 t.	125 mL	
8 oz.	1 c.	16 T.	48 t.	250 mL	
2 lb.					1 kg

Keep in mind that this is not an exact conversion, but generally may be used for food measurement.

GUIDE TO PAN SIZES

Baking Pans

Customary	Metric	Holds
8-inch pie	20-cm pie	600 mL
9-inch pie	23-cm pie	1 L
10-inch pie	25-cm pie	1.3 L
8-inch round	20-cm round	1 L
9-inch round	23-cm round	1.5 L
8-inch square	20-cm square	2 L
9-inch square	23-cm square	2.5 L
9 x 5 x 2-inch loaf	23 x 13 x 5-cm loaf	2 L
9-inch tube	23-cm tube	3 L
10-inch tube	25-cm tube	3 L
13 x 9 x 2-inch	33 x 23 x 5-cm	3.5 L
14 x 10-inch cookie tin	35 x 25-cm cookie tin	
15½ x 10½ x 1-inch	39 x 25 x 3-cm	
jelly-roll	jelly-roll	

COOKING PANS AND CASSEROLES

Customary:	Metric:
1 quart	1 L
2 quart	2 L
3 quart	3 L

OVEN COOKING GUIDES

Follow this guide for oven temperature:

Fahrenheit °F	Oven heat	Celsius °C
250–275°	very slow	120–135°
300–325°	slow	150–165°
350–375°	moderate	175–190°
400–425°	hot	200–220°
450–475°	very hot	230–245°
475–500°	hottest	250–290°

Use this meat thermometer probe guide to check the meat's internal temperature:

Fahrenheit °F	Desired Doneness		Celsius °C
140°	Beef:	rare	60°
150°		medium	65°
170°		well done	75°
160°	Lamb:	medium	70°
170°		well done	75°
180°	Veal:	well done	80°
180°	Pork:	well done	80°
185°	Poultry:	well done	85°

SPICES AND HERBS

Allspice: Cinnamon, ginger, nutmeg flavor; used in breads, pastries, jellies, jams, pickles.

Anise: Licorice flavor; used in candies, breads, fruit, wine, liqueurs.

Basil: Sweet-strong flavor; used in meat, cheese, egg, tomato dishes.

Bay Leaf: Sweet flavor; used in meat, fish, vegetable dishes.

Celery: Unique, pleasantly bitter flavor; used in anything not sweet.

Chili Powder: Hot, pungent flavor; used in Mexican, Spanish dishes.

Chive: Light onion flavor; used in anything where onion should be delicate.

Cinnamon: Pungent, sweet flavor; used in pastries, breads, pickles, wine, beer, liqueurs.

Clove: Pungent, sweet flavor; used for ham, sauces, pastries, puddings, fruit, wine, liqueurs.

Coriander: Butter-lemon flavor; used for pork, cookies, cakes, pies, puddings, fruit, wine and liqueur punches.

Garlic: Strong, aromatic flavor; used in Italian, French, and many meat dishes.

Ginger: Strong, pungent flavor; used in anything sweet, plus with beer, brandy, liqueurs.

Marjoram: Sweet, semi-pungent flavor; used in poultry, lamb, egg, vegetable dishes.

Nutmeg: Sweet, nutty flavor; used in pastries, puddings, vegetables.

Oregano: Sweet, pungent flavor; used in meat, pasta, vegetable dishes.

Paprika: Light, sweet flavor; used in salads, vegetables, poultry, fish, egg dishes; often used to brighten bland-colored casseroles or entrées.

Rosemary: Fresh, sweet flavor; used in soups, meat, and vegetable dishes.

Sage: Pungent, bitter flavor; used in stuffings, sausages, some cheese dishes.

Thyme: Pungent, semi-bitter flavor; used in salty dishes or soups.

Woodruff: Sweet vanilla flavor; used in wines, punches.

Note: Metric equivalents for the stronger spices and herbs vary for each recipe to allow for individual effectiveness at convenient measurements.

FLAVORINGS AND EXTRACTS

Orange, lime, and lemon peel give vegetables, pastries, and puddings a fresh, clean flavor; liqueur flavors, such as brandy or rum, give cakes and other desserts a company flare. Choose from the following to add some zip without calories:

Almond
Anise (Licorice)
Apricot
Banana Crème
Blackberry
Black Walnut
Blueberry
Brandy
Burnt Sugar
Butter
Butternut

Butter Rum
Cherry
Clove
Coconut
Grape
Hazelnut
Lemon
Lime
Mint
Orange

Pecan
Peppermint
Pineapple
Raspberry
Rum
Sassafras
Sherry
Strawberry
Vanilla
Walnut

APPETIZERS

Fruit Dip

8	ounces plain lo-cal yogurt	240 g
4	tablespoons lo-cal preserves	60 mL
½	teaspoon ground allspice	2 mL
½	teaspoon lemon juice	2 mL

Combine all ingredients. Whip until fluffy. Chill thoroughly.

YIELD: 1 cup (250 mL)
EXCHANGE: 1 milk
CALORIES: 192

Onion Dip

4	ounces plain lo-cal yogurt	120 g
¼	cup onions (finely chopped)	60 mL
1	teaspoon lemon juice	5 mL
1	tablespoon parsley	15 mL
	dash hot pepper sauce, horseradish, salt, pepper	

Combine all ingredients. Chill thoroughly.

YIELD: ¾ cup (185 mL)
EXCHANGE: ½ milk, ½ vegetable
CALORIES: 72

Shrimp Dip

5	small shrimp	5 small
½	teaspoon Worcestershire sauce	2 mL
1	teaspoon lemon juice	5 mL
4	ounces plain lo-cal yogurt	120 g
¼	cup Chili Sauce (page 141)	60 mL

Crush shrimp. Sprinkle with Worcestershire sauce and lemon juice. Combine yogurt and Chili Sauce. Add crushed shrimp; stir to blend. Chill.

YIELD: ¾ cup (185 mL)
EXCHANGE: 1 meat, ½ milk
CALORIES: 108

Avocado Crisps

1	very ripe avocado	1
1	teaspoon lemon juice	5 mL
1	teaspoon grated onion	5 mL
1	teaspoon onion salt	5 mL
1	teaspoon paprika	5 mL
½	teaspoon marjoram	2 mL
	thin crackers	

Peel and mash avocado. Add remaining ingredients. Beat until smooth. Spread thinly on crackers.

YIELD: 45 servings
EXCHANGE 5 SERVINGS: 1 bread, 1 fat
CALORIES 5 SERVINGS: 108

Stuffed Celery

2	5-inch stalks celery	2 12.5-cm
1	tablespoon cream cheese (softened)	15 mL
¼	teaspoon onion powder	1 mL
	dash paprika	
	salt and pepper to taste	

Thoroughly rinse and drain celery. Combine cream cheese, onion powder, and paprika. Blend until smooth and creamy. Add salt and pepper. Fill celery stalks. Chill.

YIELD: 1 serving
EXCHANGE: 1 fat
CALORIES: 50

Cheese Appetizers

4	ounces cheddar cheese (shredded)	120 g
2	tablespoons margarine	30 mL
½	cup flour	125 mL
1	teaspoon onion (grated)	5 mL
½	teaspoon salt	2 mL
¼	teaspoon pepper	1 mL

Blend cheese and margarine until smooth. Add flour, onion, salt, and pepper. Stir until smooth. Shape dough into a roll, 1¼ inch (3 cm) in diameter. Wrap in plastic wrap or aluminum foil. Chill. Cut into ¼-inch (6-mm) slices. Bake at 400° F (200° C) for 8 minutes.

YIELD: 24 servings
EXCHANGE 1 SERVING: ½ fat, ¼ bread
CALORIES 1 SERVING: 37

Cucumbers in Yogurt

1	cucumber	1
1	small onion	1 small
1	teaspoon salt	5 mL
½	teaspoon garlic powder	2 mL
1	teaspoon lemon juice	5 mL
½	teaspoon marjoram	2 mL
8	ounces lo-cal yogurt	240 g

Peel and thinly slice cucumber and onion. Sprinkle with salt. Allow to rest 15 minutes. Drain and pat dry. Combine garlic powder, lemon juice, marjoram, and yogurt; mix thoroughly. Fold in sliced cucumber and onion. Chill.

YIELD: 2 cups (500 mL)
EXCHANGE: 1 milk
CALORIES: 100

Summer Chicken Canapés

4	ounces ground cooked chicken	120 g
2	tablespoons margarine (softened)	30 mL
¼	teaspoon dry mustard	1 mL
½	teaspoon meat tenderizer	2 mL
½	teaspoon salt	2 mL
⅛	teaspoon pepper	½ mL
⅛-inch thick cucumber slices		3-m thick

Combine chicken, margarine, dry mustard, meat tenderizer, salt, and pepper. Mix thoroughly. Chill. To make canapé: Place 1 teaspoon (5 mL) of chicken mixture in center of cucumber slice.

YIELD: 24 servings
EXCHANGE 2 SERVINGS: ½ fat
CALORIES 2 SERVINGS: 28

Garlic Bites

1	slice white bread	1 slice
2	teaspoons lo-cal margarine	10 mL
¼	teaspoon garlic powder	1 mL

Remove crust from bread; cut bread into ¼-inch (6-mm) cubes. Melt margarine in small pan. Add garlic powder and heat until sizzling. Add bread cubes; sauté, tossing frequently until brown. Drain and cool.

YIELD: 2 servings
EXCHANGE 1 SERVING: ½ bread, 1 fat
CALORIES 1 SERVING: 79

Liver Paste

3	ounces chicken livers	90 g
1	tablespoon onion (finely chopped)	15 mL
1	egg (hard cooked)	1
2	teaspoons margarine	10 mL
1	tablespoon evaporated milk (regular or skim)	15 mL
	salt and pepper to taste	

Boil chicken livers and onion in small amount of water until tender. Drain. Finely chop the egg. Mash livers, onion, egg, and margarine until well blended. Add milk; blend thoroughly. Add salt and pepper.

YIELD: 24 servings, 1 teaspoon (5 mL) each
EXCHANGE 3 SERVINGS: ½ medium-fat meat
CALORIES 3 SERVINGS: 39

Smoked Salmon Canapés

8	ounces smoked salmon	240 g
3	ounces cream cheese	90 g
½	teaspoon lemon juice	2 mL
1	teaspoon milk	5 mL
	dash thyme, sage, salt, pepper	

Place smoked salmon in blender. Blend until fine. Combine cream cheese, lemon juice, and milk. Stir to make a paste. Add seasonings. Mix well. Add salmon; blend thoroughly. Roll into 22 balls. Chill.

YIELD: 22 servings
EXCHANGE 2 SERVINGS: 1 meat
CALORIES 2 SERVINGS: 68

Swiss Morsels

8	ounces Swiss cheese (grated)	240 g
4	ounces ham (grated)	120 g
2	tablespoons margarine (softened)	30 mL
¼	teaspoon thyme	1 mL

Combine all ingredients; mix thoroughly. Shape 2 teaspoons (10 mL) of mixture into a ball. Repeat with remaining mixture.

YIELD: 34 servings
EXCHANGE 1 SERVING: ½ high-fat meat
CALORIES 1 SERVING: 51

Hors d'Oeuvre Spreads

YIELD: ¼ cup (60 mL) spread for 24 crackers or ½ teaspoon (2 mL)
     per cracker

EXCHANGE PER SERVING: ½ fat plus cracker EXCHANGE

Use one of the following as a spread for 24 small crackers:

ANCHOVY

| 1 | ounce anchovy fillets | 30 g |
| ¼ | cup lo-cal margarine | 60 mL |

Rinse fillets in cold water; pat dry. Grind or chop fine; blend with margarine. Allow to rest.

EXCHANGE ¼ CUP (60 mL): 12 fat, 1 meat
CALORIES ¼ CUP (60 mL): 250

CAVIAR

| 2 | tablespoons caviar | 30 mL |
| ¼ | cup lo-cal margarine | 60 mL |

Combine caviar and margarine. Refrigerate overnight.

EXCHANGE ¼ CUP (60 mL): 12 fat, 1 meat
CALORIES ¼ CUP (60 mL): 280

CRABMEAT

| 2 | tablespoons crabmeat | 30 mL |
| ¼ | cup lo-cal margarine | 60 mL |

Crush crabmeat; blend with margarine. Refrigerate overnight.

EXCHANGE ¼ CUP (60 mL): 12 fat, ½ meat
CALORIES ¼ CUP (60 mL): 230

GARLIC

¼	teaspoon garlic	1 mL
¼	cup lo-cal margarine	60 mL
	dash salt	

Blend ingredients together.

EXCHANGE ¼ CUP (60 mL): 12 fat
CALORIES ¼ CUP (60 mL): 200

HERB

	dash each marjoram, oregano, onion (chopped), salt, pepper	
¼	cup lo-cal margarine	60 mL

Blend ingredients together; allow to rest at room temperature 2 hours.

EXCHANGE ¼ CUP (60 mL): 2 fat
CALORIES ¼ CUP (60 mL): 200

HORSERADISH

1	tablespoon horseradish (grated)	15 mL
1	teaspoon parsley (chopped)	5 mL
¼	cup lo-cal margarine	60 mL

Blend ingredients together; refrigerate overnight.

EXCHANGE ¼ CUP (60 mL): 12 fat
CALORIES ¼ CUP (60 mL): 200

LEMON

1	teaspoon lemon juice	5 mL
¼	teaspoon parsley	1 mL
¼	cup lo-cal margarine	60 mL
	dash salt	

Blend ingredients together.

EXCHANGE ¼ CUP (60 mL): 12 fat

MUSTARD

| 2 | teaspoons Dijon mustard | 10 mL |
| ¼ | cup margarine | 60 mL |

Blend ingredients together.

EXCHANGE ¼ CUP (60 mL): 12 fat
CALORIES ¼ CUP (60 mL): 200

Note: Exchange and calorie figures above do not include crackers.

Spreads may be topped with 1 teaspoon (5 mL):

Chicken	Salami	Crabmeat
Chicken liver	Sausage	Lobster
Ham	Tuna	

EXCHANGE TO ADD 6 CRACKERS: 1 meat, 1 bread

| Bacon | Avocado |

EXCHANGE TO ADD 5 CRACKERS: 1 fat, 1 bread

Cauliflower	Mushrooms	Green pepper
Celery	Onion	Radish
Cucumber	Parsley	Tomato flesh

SOUPS AND STEWS

Chicken Broth

2	pound hen (cut up)	1 kg
½	medium stalk celery (chopped)	½ medium
8–10	green onions (chopped)	8 to 10
2	tablespoons parsley (chopped)	30 mL
2	teaspoons salt	10 mL
1	teaspoon thyme	5 mL
1	teaspoon marjoram	5 mL
½	teaspoon pepper	2 mL

Wash chicken pieces; place in large kettle. Cover with 2 quarts (2 L) water; bring to a boil, cover and cook 1 hour or until chicken is tender. Add remaining ingredients; simmer 1 hour. Remove chicken; strain broth. Refrigerate broth overnight. Remove all fat from surface before reheating broth.

YIELD: 2 quarts (2 L) broth
EXCHANGE: Negligible
CALORIES: Negligible

Beef Broth

3–4	pounds beef soup bones or chuck roast	1½ to 2 kg
½	stalk celery (chopped)	½ stalk
3	carrots (sliced)	3
1	medium onion (chopped)	1 medium
½	green pepper (chopped)	½
2	bay leaves	2
½	teaspoon each thyme, marjoram, paprika, pepper	2 mL each
2	teaspoons salt	10 mL

Place beef in large kettle; cover with 2 quarts (2 L) water. Bring to a boil; cover and cook 2 hours or until meat is tender. Add remaining ingredients; simmer 1 hour. Remove beef; strain broth. Refrigerate broth overnight. Remove all fat from surface before reheating broth.

YIELD: 2 quarts (2 L) broth
EXCHANGE: Negligible
CALORIES: Negligible

Broth with Vegetables

Cook ½ cup (125 mL) vegetables or combination of vegetables in boiling salted water; drain. Add to hot broth just before serving.

MICROWAVE: Add ½ cup (125 mL) vegetables (no water needed). Cook on High for 3 minutes. Add to hot broth just before serving.

YIELD: ½ cup (125 mL)
EXCHANGE: ½ vegetable
CALORIES: 18

Broth with Noodles

Cook ¼ cup (60 mL) noodles or broken spaghetti in boiling salted water; drain. Add to hot broth just before serving.

MICROWAVE: Add ¼ cup (60 mL) noodles or pasta to 2 cups (500 mL) boiling salted water. Cook on High for 3 minutes. Hold 3 minutes. Drain. Add to hot broth just before serving.

YIELD: ½ cup (125 mL)
EXCHANGE: 1 bread
CALORIES: 68

Broth Italiano

⅛	cup vermicelli (broken)	30 mL
1	cup broth	250 mL
1	ounce thinly sliced prosciutto (shredded)	30 g
⅛	teaspoon garlic powder	½ mL
⅛	teaspoon marjoram	½ mL
1	tablespoon Parmesan cheese (grated)	15 mL

Cook vermicelli in boiling salted water; drain and rinse. Bring broth to a boil. Add prosciutto, garlic powder, and marjoram. Simmer 5 minutes. Add vermicelli. Pour into bowl. Sprinkle Parmesan cheese over top.

YIELD: 1½ cups (375 mL)
EXCHANGE: ½ bread, 1 medium-fat meat
CALORIES: 107

Broth Madeira

Add 1 tablespoon (15 mL) Madeira to 1 cup (250 mL) broth. Bring just to a boil. Garnish with lemon slice and fresh chopped parsley.

MICROWAVE: Add 1 tablespoon (15 mL) Madeira to 1 cup (250 mL) broth. Cook on High for 2 minutes. Garnish with lemon slice and fresh chopped parsley.

> YIELD: 1 cup (250 mL)
> EXCHANGE: Negligible
> CALORIES: Negligible

Vegetable Broth

1	cup onion (chopped)	250 mL
2	cups carrots (diced)	500 mL
1	cup celery (chopped)	250 mL
2	cups spinach (cut in small pieces)	500 mL
2	cups tomato (peeled and chopped)	500 mL
1	bay leaf	1
2	tablespoons parsley or parsley flakes	30 mL
½	teaspoon thyme	2 mL
1	blade mace	1 blade
¼	teaspoon garlic or garlic powder	1 mL
1	tablespoon Worcestershire	15 mL
	salt to taste	

Place vegetables in large kettle. Cover with 2 to 3 quarts (2 to 3 L) water. Bring to a boil; reduce heat and simmer for 2 hours. Stir frequently. Add seasonings. Simmer 1 hour. Strain. Add water to make 2 quarts (2 L).

> YIELD: 2 quarts (2 L) broth
> EXCHANGE: Negligible
> CALORIES: Negligible

Broth Orientale

2	tablespoons rice	30 mL
1½	cups vegetable broth	375 mL
1	tablespoon celery (thinly sliced)	15 mL
½	teaspoon onion (finely chopped)	2 mL
1	tablespoon bean sprouts	15 mL
1	water chestnut (thinly sliced)	1
	salt to taste	

Add rice to cold vegetable broth; bring to boil. Reduce heat; simmer 20 minutes. Add celery, onion, bean sprouts, and water chestnut; simmer 10 minutes. Add salt.

MICROWAVE: Add rice to cold broth; heat to a boil. Cover. Hold 15 minutes. Add remaining ingredients, except salt. Cook 3 minutes. Hold 5 minutes. Add salt.

YIELD: 1¼ cups (310 mL)
EXCHANGE: ⅛ bread, ⅛ vegetable
CALORIES: 11

Tomato Beef Bouillon

2	tablespoons margarine	30 mL
¼	cup onion (chopped)	60 mL
46	ounces tomato juice	1½ L
2	cans beef broth **OR**	2 cans
2½	cups homemade beef broth	625 mL
1	bay leaf	1
1	teaspoon salt	5 mL
½	teaspoon pepper	2 mL

Heat margarine in a large saucepan. Add onion and cook until tender. Add tomato juice, beef broth (canned or homemade), bay leaf, salt, and pepper; heat thoroughly. DO NOT BOIL. Remove bay leaf. Ladle into warm bowls.

ADDED TOUCH: Top each serving with 1 teaspoon (5 mL) grated American cheese.

YIELD: 8 servings, 1 cup (250 mL) each
EXCHANGE 1 SERVING: ¼ vegetable, 1 fat
CALORIES 1 SERVING: 58

Greek Egg Lemon Soup

2	quarts chicken broth	2 L
3	eggs (separated)	3
	juice of 1 lemon	

Bring broth to a boil in saucepan. Beat egg whites until stiff. Add egg yolks. Beat slowly until mixture is a light yellow. Add lemon juice gradually, beating constantly. Pour small amount of chicken broth into egg mixture. Pour egg mixture into hot broth, beating constantly.

YIELD: 8 servings, 1 cup (250 mL) each
EXCHANGE 1 SERVING: ¼ high-fat meat
CALORIES 1 SERVING: 27

Quick Egg Soup

1½	cups boiling water	375 mL
1	cube vegetable bouillon	1 cube
1	egg	1

Dissolve bouillon cube in boiling water; remove from heat. Beat egg; blend into vegetable broth. Reheat slowly. DO NOT BOIL.

YIELD: 1½ cups (375 mL)
EXCHANGE: 1 medium-fat meat
CALORIES: 80

German Cabbage Soup

2	ounces ground beef round	60 g
2	tablespoons onion (grated)	30 mL
	dash mustard, soy sauce, salt, pepper	
1	tablespoon dry red wine	15 mL
1¼	cups beef broth	310 mL
2	large cabbage leaves (cut in pieces)	2 large
½	medium tomato (cubed)	½ medium
½	teaspoon fresh parsley (chopped)	2 mL

Combine ground round, onion, mustard, soy sauce, salt, and pepper; mix thoroughly. Form into tiny meatballs. Add wine to broth; bring to a boil. Add meatballs to broth, one at a time. Bring to boil again. Cook meatballs 5 minutes; remove to soup bowl. Add cabbage and tomatoes to broth. Simmer 5 minutes. Pour over meatballs. Garnish with parsley.

YIELD: 1 ½ cups (375 mL)
EXCHANGE: 1 ½ medium-fat meat, ½ vegetable
CALORIES: 55

Borscht

	16-ounce can beets with juice	500-g can
2	tablespoons sugar replacement	30 mL
¾	teaspoon salt	3 mL
3	tablespoons lemon juice	45 mL
½	teaspoon thyme	2 mL
1	egg (well beaten)	1

Purée beets in blender. Add enough water to make 1 quart (1 L). Pour into saucepan. Add sugar replacement, salt, lemon juice, and thyme; heat to a boil. Remove from heat. Add small amount of hot beet mixture to egg. Stir egg mixture into beet mixture. Return to heat; cook and stir until hot. DO NOT BOIL.

YIELD: 4 servings, 1 cup (250 mL) each
EXCHANGE 1 SERVING: 1 vegetable, ¼ high-fat meat
CALORIES 1 SERVING: 104

ADDED TOUCH: Top each serving with 1 teaspoon (5 mL) lo-cal sour cream.

French Meatball Soup

2	tablespoons rice (uncooked)	30 mL
2	ounces ground beef round	60 g
1	tablespoon egg (raw, beaten)	15 mL
1	teaspoon onion (grated)	5 mL
	dash garlic, parsley, nutmeg	
2	tablespoons dry red wine	30 mL
1¼	cups beef broth	310 mL
	salt and pepper to taste	

Add rice to 1 cup (250 mL) salted water. Boil 5 minutes; drain well. Blend rice, ground round, egg, onion, garlic, parsley, and nutmeg; form into small meatballs. Add wine to broth; bring to a boil. Drop meatballs into hot broth, one at a time. Bring to boil again; reduce heat. Simmer 20 minutes. Add salt and pepper.

MICROWAVE: Add rice to 1 cup (250 mL) salted water. Bring to a boil. Hold 5 minutes; drain well. Combine meatball ingredients as above. Bring wine and broth to a boil. Drop meatballs into hot broth, one at a time. Bring to a boil again. Set aside 10 minutes. Add salt and pepper.

YIELD: 1½ cups (375 mL)
EXCHANGE: 2 medium-fat meat, ½ bread
CALORIES: 71

Ham and Split Pea Soup

2	pounds meaty ham bone	1 kg
1	bay leaf	1
2	cups dried green split peas, soaked overnight	500 mL
1	cup onions (chopped)	250 mL
1	cup celery (cubed)	250 mL
1	cup carrots (grated)	250 mL
	salt and pepper to taste	

Cover ham bone and bay leaf with water. Simmer for 2 to 2½ hours. Remove bone and strain liquid. Refrigerate overnight. Remove lean meat from bone; set aside. Remove fat from surface of liquid. Heat liquid; add enough water to make 2½ quarts (2½ L). Add peas; simmer for 20 minutes. Remove from heat and allow to stand 1 hour. Add onions, celery, carrots, and lean pieces of ham. Add salt and pepper. Simmer for 40 minutes. Stir occasionally.

YIELD: 10 servings
EXCHANGE 1 SERVING: ½ high-fat meat, 1 vegetable
CALORIES 1 SERVING: 204

Cream of Chicken and Almond Soup

1	cup chicken broth	250 mL
1	whole clove	1
1	sprig parsley	1 sprig
½	bay leaf	½
	pinch mace	
1	tablespoon celery (sliced)	15 mL
1	tablespoon carrot (diced)	15 mL
1	teaspoon onion (diced)	5 mL
2	teaspoons stale bread crumbs	10 mL
½	ounce chicken breast (cubed)	15 g
1	teaspoon blanched almonds (crushed)	5 mL

¼	cup skim milk	60 mL
1	teaspoon flour	5 mL
	salt and pepper to taste	

Heat chicken broth, clove, parsley, bay leaf, and mace to a boil; remove from heat. Allow to rest 10 minutes; strain. Add celery, carrot, onion, bread crumbs, chicken, and almonds to seasoned chicken broth; simmer 20 minutes. Blend in skim milk and flour. Remove soup from heat; add milk mixture. Return to heat. Simmer (do not boil) 3 to 5 minutes. Add salt and pepper.

YIELD: 1½ cups (375 mL)
EXCHANGE: ½ lean meat, 1 vegetable, ¼ milk
CALORIES: 89

Crab Chowder

1	cup milk	250 mL
1	teaspoon flour	5 mL
¼	cup water	60 mL
¼	cup cooked crabmeat (flaked)	60 mL
3	tablespoons mushroom pieces	45 mL
3	tablespoons asparagus pieces	45 mL
	salt and pepper to taste	

Blend milk, flour, and water thoroughly; pour into saucepan. Add crabmeat, mushrooms, and asparagus. Cook over low heat until slightly thickened. Add salt and pepper.

YIELD: 1 cup (250 mL)
EXCHANGE: 1 milk, 1 vegetable, 1 lean meat
CALORIES: 150

Clam Chowder

1	slice bacon	1 slice
1½	cups fish or vegetable broth	375 mL
2	tablespoons carrot (diced)	30 mL
1	tablespoon onion (diced)	15 mL
1	tablespoon celery (diced)	15 mL
1	large tomato (diced)	1 large
1	medium potato (diced)	1 medium
	dash thyme, rosemary, salt, pepper	
1	teaspoon flour	5 mL
¼	cup water	60 mL
1	ounce clams	30 g

Cook bacon until crisp; drain and crumble. Combine broth, carrot, onion, celery, tomato, potato, and seasonings. Simmer until vegetables are tender. Blend flour and water; stir into chowder. Reduce heat. Add clams and crumbled bacon. Heat to thicken slightly.

MICROWAVE: Combine vegetables with broth and seasonings; cover. Cook on High for 4 minutes, or until vegetables are tender. Add flour–water mixture. Cook 30 seconds; stir. Add clams and bacon; stir. Cook 30 seconds. Hold 3 minutes.

YIELD: 2 cups (500 mL)
EXCHANGE: 1 lean meat, 1 fat, 1 vegetable, 1 bread
CALORIES: 200

Fish Chowder

2	cups water	500 mL
3	ounces bullhead fillet	90 g
1	medium potato (diced)	1 medium
3	tablespoons onion (diced)	45 mL
3	tablespoons celery (diced)	45 mL
2	tablespoons carrot (diced)	30 mL
1	medium tomato (diced)	1 medium
	salt and pepper to taste	

Combine all ingredients in saucepan. Heat to a boil; cover and reduce heat. Simmer 1 to 1½ hours.

YIELD: 3 servings, 1 cup (250 mL) each
EXCHANGE 1 SERVING: 1 medium-fat meat, ½ vegetable, ½ bread
CALORIES 1 SERVING: 81

Oyster Stew

1	teaspoon flour	5 mL
1	tablespoon celery (minced)	15 mL
1	teaspoon salt	5 mL
	dash Worcestershire sauce, soy sauce	
1	tablespoon water	15 mL
1	ounce oysters (with liquid)	30 g
1	teaspoon butter	5 mL
1	cup skim milk	250 mL

Blend flour, celery, seasoning, and water in saucepan; add oysters with liquid and butter. Simmer over low heat until edges of oysters curl. Remove from heat; add skim milk. Reheat over low heat. Add extra salt if desired.

YIELD: 1½ cups (375 mL)
EXCHANGE: 1 lean meat, 1 milk, ¼ bread
CALORIES: 220

Kidney Stew

2	ounces beef kidney (cooked)	60 g
1½	cups beef broth	375 mL
3	tablespoons leek (chopped)	45 mL
1	slice bacon (cooked and drained)	1 slice
¼	cup mushrooms	60 mL
3	tablespoons green pepper (sliced)	45 mL
	dash parsley, thyme, tarragon, salt, pepper	

Heat all ingredients to a boil. Reduce heat and simmer until green pepper slices are tender.

YIELD: 1 ½ cups (375 mL)
EXCHANGE: 2 lean meat, 1 fat
CALORIES: 130

Pizza Stew

1	ounce Canadian bacon	30 g
1½	cups Tomato Sauce (page 140)	375 mL
¼	cup water	60 mL
2	tablespoons onion (chopped)	30 mL
1	tablespoon mushroom pieces	15 mL
1	tablespoon black olives (pitted and chopped)	15 mL
1	tablespoon celery (chopped)	15 mL
1	tablespoon green pepper (chopped)	15 mL
	dash oregano, garlic powder, salt to taste	
½	cup elbow macaroni (cooked)	125 mL

Fry Canadian bacon; drain and cut away any fat. Heat Tomato Sauce and water to a boil. Add bacon, vegetables, and seasonings. Cook until vegetables are tender. Add macaroni; reheat.

YIELD: 2¼ cups (560 mL)
EXCHANGE: 1 high-fat meat, 1 bread, 1 vegetable
CALORIES: 275

Bean Stew

1	tablespoon pinto beans	15 mL
1	tablespoon northern beans	15 mL
1	tablespoon lentils	15 mL
1	cup beef broth	250 mL
1	tablespoon carrot (sliced)	15 mL
1	tablespoon hominy	15 mL
1	teaspoon onion (diced)	5 mL
½	teaspoon green chilies (chopped)	2 mL
	dash garlic powder, oregano, salt, pepper	

Boil beans and lentils in beef broth for 10 minutes, covered. Allow to stand 1 to 2 hours, or overnight. Place softened beans and remaining ingredients in baking dish. Bake at 350° F (175° C) for 45 minutes to 1 hour, or until ingredients are tender.

MICROWAVE: Place beans and lentils in beef broth; cover. Cook on High for 5 minutes. Allow to stand 1 to 2 hours or overnight. Add remaining ingredients. Cook on Medium for 10 to 15 minutes, or until ingredients are tender.

YIELD: 1½ cups (375 mL)
EXCHANGE: 1 lean meat, 2 bread
CALORIES: 225

Zucchini Meatball Stew

1	ounce ground beef	30 g
½	cup ground zucchini	125 mL
1	teaspoon onion (finely chopped)	5 mL
1	egg	1
¼	cup rice (uncooked)	60 mL
	dash oregano, cumin, garlic salt, pepper	
1	cup beef broth	250 mL
1	large tomato (diced)	1 large
1	teaspoon parsley (chopped)	5 mL
	salt and pepper to taste	

Combine ground beef, zucchini, onion, egg, rice, and seasonings; mix thoroughly. Shape into small meatballs. Combine beef broth, tomato, and parsley in saucepan; heat to boil. Drop meatballs into hot broth, one at a time. Cover and simmer 30 to 40 minutes. Add salt and pepper.

MICROWAVE: Cook beef broth, tomato, and parsley on High for 3 minutes, covered. Drop meatballs into broth. Cook on High 5 minutes. Hold 10 minutes. Add salt and pepper.

YIELD: 1¾ cups (435 mL)
EXCHANGE: 2 medium-fat meat, 1 vegetable, 1 bread
CALORIES: 203

Chicken Giblet Stew

3	ounces chicken giblets	90 g
2	cups water	500 mL
¼	teaspoon thyme	1 mL
¼	bay leaf	¼
⅛	teaspoon parsley (crushed)	½ mL
	salt and pepper to taste	
3	tablespoons potatoes (diced)	45 mL
2	tablespoons onion (diced)	30 mL
2	tablespoons celery (diced)	30 mL
2	tablespoons green beans (sliced)	30 mL
2	tablespoons carrots (diced)	30 mL
2	tablespoons peas	30 mL
1	teaspoon flour	5 mL
¼	cup water	60 mL

Remove center muscle of giblets. Place the 2 cups water, giblets, and seasonings in saucepan; cover. Heat to a boil; reduce heat and simmer until giblets are tender, about 1 hour. Add extra water to make about 2 cups (500 mL) liquid. Remove bay leaf. Add vegetables; reheat and cook until vegetables are tender. Blend flour with the ¼ cup water. Blend into stew. Cook to desired thickness.

YIELD: 3 servings, 1 cup (250 mL) each
EXCHANGE 1 SERVING: 1 lean meat, 1 bread, 1 vegetable
CALORIES 1 SERVING: 120

Pepper Pot

(Leftovers may be used)

2	ounces lean pork, cut in 1-inch (2.5-cm) cubes	60 g
1	ounce beef, cut in 1-inch (2.5-cm) cubes	30 g
1	ounce chicken, cut in 1-inch (2.5-cm) cubes	30 g
¼	cup carrot pieces	60 mL
¼	cup onion slices	60 mL
¼	cup celery pieces	60 mL
¼	cup potatoes (cubed)	60 mL
½	cup water	125 mL
1	teaspoon flour	5 mL
	dash curry powder, garlic powder, salt, pepper	

Brown pork and beef cubes slowly in frying pan. Add chicken cubes for last few minutes; drain. Place meat, carrots, onions, celery, and potatoes in individual baking dish. Combine water, flour, and seasonings in screw-top jar; shake to blend well. Pour over meat mixture. Cover tightly and bake at 350° F (175° C) for 45 minutes to 1 hour, or until meat is tender and gravy has thickened.

MICROWAVE: Reduce water to ¼ cup (60 mL). Cover. Cook on High for 10 minutes. Hold 5 minutes.

YIELD: 1 serving
EXCHANGE: 4 high-fat meat, 1 vegetable, 1 bread
CALORIES: 418

Stefado

1	stick cinnamon	1 stick
1	bay leaf	1
5	whole cloves	5 whole
12	ounces beef roast (cubed)	360 g
	salt and pepper to taste	
1	teaspoon margarine	5 mL
1½	cups onions (sliced)	375 mL
3	medium tomatoes (peeled and cubed)	3 medium
½	cup red wine	125 mL
1	teaspoon brown sugar replacement	5 mL
2	tablespoons raisins	30 mL
1	cup water	250 mL
1	garlic clove (crushed)	1

Place cinnamon, bay leaf, and cloves in small cheesecloth bag. Combine with remaining ingredients in soup kettle; cook 1 to 1½ hours until meat is tender. Remove spice bag before serving.

MICROWAVE: Same as above. Cook on High 15 to 20 minutes.

YIELD: 3 servings, 1 cup (250 mL) each
EXCHANGE 1 SERVING: 4 high-fat meat, 1 vegetable
CALORIES 1 SERVING: 430

CASSEROLES AND ONE-DISH MEALS

Beef Stroganoff

3	ounces lean beef (cubed)	90 g
1	teaspoon margarine	5 mL
½	onion (cut into large pieces)	½
¼	teaspoon garlic (minced)	1 mL
2	tablespoons mushroom pieces	30 mL
½	cup condensed cream of mushroom soup	125 mL
1	tablespoon lo-cal sour cream	15 mL
1	teaspoon ketchup	5 mL
	dash Worcestershire sauce, ground bay leaf, salt, pepper	
1	cup noodles (cooked)	250 mL

Brown beef cubes in margarine. Add onion, garlic, and mushrooms. Cook over low heat until onion is partially cooked; remove from heat. Combine condensed soup, sour cream, ketchup, and seasonings; blend well. Pour over beef mixture; heat thoroughly. Do not boil. Serve over noodles.

YIELD: 1 serving
EXCHANGE: 3 high-fat meat, 2½ bread
CALORIES: 470

Packaged Steak Supper

3	ounces beef minute steak	90 g
1	small potato	1 small
2	tablespoons carrot (sliced)	30 mL
2	tablespoons onion (sliced)	30 mL
2	tablespoons celery (sliced)	30 mL
2	large tomato slices	2 large
	salt and pepper to taste	

Place steak on large piece of aluminum foil. Layer vegetables in order given. Add salt and pepper. Wrap in foil, sealing ends securely. Bake at 350° F (175° C) for 1 hour.

MICROWAVE: Place in plastic wrap. Cook on High for 10 minutes.

YIELD: 1 serving
EXCHANGE: 3 medium-fat meat, 1 bread, ½ vegetable
CALORIES: 375

Quick Kabobs

2	ounces cooked roast beef, cut in 1-inch cubes	60 g
6	1-inch (2.5-cm) green pepper squares	6
6	cherry tomatoes	6
6	1-inch (2.5-cm) zucchini cubes	6
6	unsweetened pineapple chunks	6
2	tablespoons lo-cal French dressing	30 mL

Alternate beef, vegetables, and fruit on 2 skewers. Brush with 1 tablespoon (15 mL) of the French dressing. Broil 5 to 6 inches (12.5

to 15 cm) from heat for 8 minutes. Brush with remaining French dressing. Broil 4 minutes longer.

YIELD: 1 serving (2 kabobs)
EXCHANGE: 2 medium-fat meat, 1 vegetable, 1 fruit
CALORIES: 150

Beef and Rice Casserole

3	ounces ground beef	90 g
1	tablespoon onion (chopped)	15 mL
1	tablespoon celery (chopped)	15 mL
¾	cup condensed chicken gumbo soup	185 mL
¼	cup water	60 mL
½	cup rice (uncooked)	125 mL
¼	cup condensed cream of mushroom soup	60 mL
	salt and pepper to taste	

Combine ground beef, onion, and celery with a small amount of water in a saucepan. Boil until onion is tender; drain. Combine condensed chicken gumbo soup, water, and rice. Simmer until all moisture is absorbed. Mix beef mixture, rice, and mushroom soup; pour into a small greased casserole dish. Add salt and pepper. Bake at 350° F (175° C) for 25 minutes.

MICROWAVE: Cook on Medium for 8 to 10 minutes.

YIELD: 1 serving
EXCHANGE: 3 high-fat meat, 2 bread
CALORIES: 380

German Goulash

3	ounces lean ground beef	90 g
1	teaspoon onion (chopped)	5 mL
1	tablespoon green pepper (chopped)	15 mL
1	tablespoon celery (chopped)	15 mL
¼	bay leaf (crushed)	¼
½	cup kidney beans (cooked)	125 mL
½	cup elbow macaroni (cooked)	125 mL
¼	cup carrot (sliced)	60 mL
	salt and pepper to taste	

Brown ground beef, onion, green pepper, and celery over low heat; drain. Add crushed bay leaf, kidney beans, macaroni, and carrots; mix gently. Add salt and pepper. Pour into casserole dish; cover. Bake at 350° F (175° C) for 40 minutes.

MICROWAVE: Cook on Medium for 7 minutes.

YIELD: 1 serving
EXCHANGE: 3 medium-fat meat, 2½ bread
CALORIES: 413

Stuffed Peppers

1	green pepper	1
2	tablespoons rice	30 mL
2	ounces lean ground beef	60 g
1	egg	1
1	teaspoon onion flakes	5 mL
1	tablespoon mushrooms (finely chopped)	15 mL
	salt and pepper to taste	
1	teaspoon Tomato Sauce (page 140) 5 mL	

Cut green pepper in half, lengthwise. Remove membrane and seeds; rinse, drain, and reserve shells. Boil rice with ½ cup (125 mL) of water for 5 minutes; drain. Combine ground beef, rice, egg, onion flakes, and mushrooms; blend thoroughly. Add salt and pepper. Fill green pepper cavities with beef mixture; top with Tomato Sauce. Place in baking dish; cover. Bake at 350° F (175° C) for 20 to 25 minutes.

MICROWAVE: Cook on High for 10 minutes.

YIELD: 1 serving
EXCHANGE: 3 medium-fat meat, 1 bread, 1 vegetable
CALORIES: 255

Lasagne

2	ounces ground beef	60 g
1	tablespoon onion (chopped)	15 mL
½	cup Tomato Sauce (page 140)	125 mL
3	tablespoons water	45 mL
¼	teaspoon garlic powder	1 mL
½	teaspoon oregano	2 mL
	salt and pepper to taste	
1½	cups lasagne noodles (cooked)	375 mL
1	ounce mozzarella cheese (grated)	30 g
1	ounce provolone cheese (grated)	30 g

Crumble beef in small amount of water; add onion. Boil until meat is cooked; drain. Blend Tomato Sauce, 3 tablespoons (45 mL) water, garlic powder, oregano, salt, and pepper. Add beef–onion mixture; stir to blend. Spread small amount of sauce into bottom of individual baking dish.

Layer noodles, sauce, mozzarella, and provolone cheese. Bake at 375° F (190° C) for 30 minutes.

MICROWAVE: Cook on High for 10 minutes.

YIELD: 1 serving
EXCHANGE: 4 high-fat meat, 3 bread
CALORIES: 485

Hamburger Pie

2	pounds lean ground beef	1 kg
½	cup cornflakes (crushed)	125 mL
¼	teaspoon garlic powder	1 mL
½	teaspoon onion (finely chopped)	2 mL
1	egg	1
	salt and pepper to taste	
2¼	cups water	560 mL
1	cup skim milk	250 mL
1	teaspoon salt	5 mL
2	cups instant mashed potatoes	500 mL
1	teaspoon margarine	5 mL

Combine ground beef, cornflakes, garlic powder, onion, and egg; mix well. Add salt and pepper. Place beef mixture in 9-inch (23-cm) pie pan. Pat to cover bottom and sides evenly. Bake at 425° F (220° C) for 30 minutes; drain off excess fat. Heat water, skim milk, and salt just to a boil; remove from heat. Add potato granules; mix thoroughly. Add margarine; blend well. Cover and allow to stand 5 minutes, or until potatoes thicken. Spread evenly over meat mixture. Return to oven and bake until potatoes are golden brown. Allow to rest 10 minutes before cutting pie into wedges.

MICROWAVE: Cover beef mixture. Cook on Medium for 10 to 12 minutes; drain. Cover with potatoes. Cook on Medium for 2 minutes. Hold 5 minutes.

YIELD: 8 servings
EXCHANGE 1 SERVING: 4 high-fat meat, 1 bread, ½ fat
CALORIES 1 SERVING: 372

Wiener-Egg Scramble

1	slice bacon	1 slice
1	teaspoon onion (chopped)	5 mL
1	wiener (sliced)	1
½	teaspoon green pepper (chopped)	2 mL
1	egg	1
1	teaspoon skim milk	5 mL
	dash Worcestershire sauce	

Cook bacon until crisp; drain bacon and remove from pan. Crumble bacon. Place bacon, onion, wiener, and green pepper in pan. Sauté on low heat until onion is tender. Beat egg with skim milk and Worcestershire sauce; pour over wiener mixture. Cook until set.

YIELD: 1 serving
EXCHANGE: 2 high-fat meat, 2 fat
CALORIES: 170

Cheese Lasagne

½	cup Tomato Sauce (page 140)	125 mL
3	tablespoons water	45 mL
1	tablespoon onion	15 mL
¼	teaspoon garlic powder	1 mL
½	teaspoon oregano	2 mL
	salt and pepper to taste	
¼	cup large curd cottage cheese	60 mL
1	egg	1
1½	cups lasagne noodles (cooked)	375 mL
2	ounces mozzarella cheese	60 g
1	tablespoon Parmesan cheese	15 mL

Combine Tomato Sauce, water, onion, garlic powder, oregano, salt, and pepper. Thoroughly blend together cottage cheese and egg. Spread small amount of sauce into bottom of individual baking dish. Alternate layers of noodles, sauce, cottage cheese mixture, and mozzarella cheese. Top with Parmesan cheese. Bake at 375° F (190° C) for 30 minutes.

MICROWAVE: Cook on High for 10 minutes.

YIELD: 1 serving
EXCHANGE: 4 medium-fat meat, 3 bread
CALORIES: 350

Clam Pilaf

2	ounces clams (minced)	60 g
½	cup rice (cooked)	125 mL
2	tablespoons onion (chopped)	30 mL
1	medium fresh tomato (peeled and cubed)	1 medium
	dash ground bay leaf, thyme, salt, pepper	
2	tablespoons grated Cheddar cheese	30 mL

Combine clams, rice, onion, tomato, and seasonings in baking dish; top with cheese. Bake at 350° F (175° C) for 25 minutes.

MICROWAVE: Combine clams, rice, onion, tomato, and seasonings. Cook on High for 5 minutes; top with cheese. Reheat on High for 1 minute.

YIELD: 1 serving
EXCHANGE: 2 lean meat, 1 bread
CALORIES: 170

Macaroni and Cheese Supreme

1	cup elbow macaroni	250 mL
11-ounce can condensed cream		
	of mushroom soup	300-g can
6	ounces cheese (shredded)	180 mL
1	teaspoon yellow mustard	5 mL
1	teaspoon salt	5 mL
	dash pepper	
2	cups cooked spinach (drained)	500 mL
12	ounces lean meat (diced)	360 g

Cook macaroni as directed on package; drain. Combine mushroom soup, cheese, mustard, salt, and pepper. Add macaroni; stir well. Spread cooked spinach on bottom of lightly greased 13 x 9-inch (33 x 23-cm) baking dish. Top with meat. Spoon macaroni mixture evenly over entire surface. Bake at 375° F (190° C) for 40 minutes. Allow to cool 15 minutes before serving.

MICROWAVE: Cook on Medium for 12 to 15 minutes. Turn dish halfway through cooking time. Allow to rest 15 minutes before serving.

YIELD: 6 servings
EXCHANGE 1 SERVING: 2 bread, 3 high-fat meat, 1 vegetable
CALORIES 1 SERVING: 287

Turkey à la King I

1	tablespoon green pepper (diced)	15 mL
2	tablespoons celery (sliced)	30 mL
¼	cup condensed cream of chicken soup	60 mL
2	tablespoons skim milk	30 mL
2	tablespoons mushrooms (chopped)	30 mL
3	ounces cooked turkey (diced)	90 g
1	tablespoon pimiento (chopped)	15 mL
	salt and pepper to taste	
2	slices bread (toasted)	2 slices

Cook green pepper and celery in boiling water until tender; drain. Blend condensed soup and skim milk. Add green pepper, celery, mushrooms, turkey, and pimiento. Add salt and pepper. Heat slightly over low heat. Cut toast into triangles; place in small bowl, tips up. Spoon turkey mixture over tips.

YIELD: 1 serving
EXCHANGE: 3 medium-fat meat, 2¼ bread, ¼ vegetable
CALORIES: 450

Turkey à la King II

¼	cup White Sauce (page 147)	60 mL
1	ounce cooked turkey (diced)	30 g
¼	cup mushroom pieces	60 mL
2	tablespoons green pepper (chopped)	30 mL
1	tablespoon stuffed green olives (chopped)	15 mL
	salt and pepper to taste	
	dough for 1 Baking Powder Biscuit (page 95)	

Heat White Sauce. Combine sauce, turkey, mushrooms, green pepper, and olives; add salt and pepper. Pour into lightly greased individual baking dish. Top with biscuit dough. Bake at 375° F (190° C) for 15 to 20 minutes, or until biscuit is golden brown.

YIELD: 1 serving
EXCHANGE: 1 medium-fat meat, 1 vegetable, 1 bread
CALORIES: 168

Chicken Gambeano

¼	cup condensed cream of chicken soup	60 mL
3	tablespoons skim milk	45 mL
¼	cup zucchini (cubed)	60 mL
¼	cup green beans	60 mL
2	ounces cooked chicken (cubed)	60 g
¼	teaspoon poultry seasoning	1 mL
	salt and pepper to taste	
1¼	cups linguine (cooked)	310 mL

Blend condensed soup and skim milk; place in saucepan. Add zucchini and green beans. Cook over medium heat until vegetables are partially tender. Add chicken and seasonings; reheat. Serve over linguine.

MICROWAVE: Blend condensed soup and skim milk in bowl. Add zucchini and green beans; cover. Cook on High for 5 to 7 minutes, or until vegetables are partially tender. Add chicken and seasonings; reheat on Medium for 4 minutes. Serve over linguine.

YIELD: 1 serving
EXCHANGE: 3 bread, 2 medium-fat meat, ½ vegetable
CALORIES: 300

Mostaccioli with Oysters

8-ounce can oysters with liquid (minced)		225 g
4-ounce can mushroom pieces		120 g
½	cup green pepper (sliced)	125 mL
1	tablespoon parsley	15 mL
1	teaspoon garlic powder	5 mL
	salt and pepper to taste	
3	cups mostaccioli noodles (cooked)	750 mL

Combine minced oysters with liquid, mushrooms, green pepper, and parsley in saucepan. Add garlic powder. Cook until green pepper is crispy tender. Add salt and pepper. Serve over mostaccioli noodles.

MICROWAVE: Combine minced oysters with liquid, mushrooms, green pepper, parsley, and garlic powder in bowl. Cook on High for 4 minutes or until green pepper is crispy tender. Add salt and pepper. Serve over mostaccioli noodles.

YIELD: 2 servings
EXCHANGE 1 SERVING: 4 lean meat, 1½ bread
CALORIES 1 SERVING: 195

Fish Noodle Special

¼	cup condensed cream of celery soup	60 mL
2	tablespoons water	30 mL
2	tablespoons mushroom pieces	30 mL
2	tablespoons onion (finely chopped)	30 mL
	dash thyme, ground rosemary, salt, pepper	
1	cup noodles (cooked)	250 mL
2	tablespoons peas	30 mL
3	ounces cooked perch (flaked)	90 g

Blend condensed soup with water. Add mushrooms, onion, and seasonings; mix thoroughly. Combine noodles, peas, and perch in small baking dish. Pour soup mixture over entire surface; toss to mix. Bake at 350° F (175° C) for 30 minutes.

MICROWAVE: Cook on High for 5 to 6 minutes.

YIELD: 1 serving
EXCHANGE: 3 lean meat, 2½ bread
CALORIES: 285

Veal Steak Parmesan

1	tablespoon flour	15 mL
1	teaspoon salt	5 mL
	dash poultry seasoning, salt, pepper, paprika	
4	ounces veal steak (cut in half)	120 g
1	teaspoon shortening	5 mL
½	cup wide noodles (cooked)	125 mL
½	cup sour cream sauce, prepared	125 mL
3	tablespoons hot water	45 mL
1	teaspoon Parmesan cheese	5 mL

Combine flour, salt, and seasonings in shaker bag. Add veal steak; shake to coat. Remove veal from bag and shake off excess flour. Heat shortening in small skillet. Brown veal on both sides; place in small baking dish. Cover with noodles. Blend sour cream sauce and hot water. Pour over noodles. Top with Parmesan cheese. Bake at 350° F (175° C) for 45 minutes, or until veal is tender.

MICROWAVE: Cover. Cook on Medium to High for 15 minutes, or until meat is tender.

YIELD: 1 serving
EXCHANGE: 4¼ medium-fat meat, 2 bread
CALORIES: 390

Kole 'n Klump

½	cup Brussels sprouts	125 mL
2	ounces lean pork cubes	60 g
	pinch caraway seeds, salt, pepper	
¼	cup potato (grated)	60 mL
¼	teaspoon onion salt	1 mL
	dash thyme, salt, pepper	

Boil Brussels sprouts, pork, caraway seeds, salt, and pepper with a small amount of water until partially cooked; drain. Place in individual baking dish. Cover with potato; sprinkle with onion salt, thyme, salt, and pepper. Cover tightly. Bake at 375° F (190° C) for 1 hour.

MICROWAVE: Cook on High for 10 to 12 minutes. Turn dish a quarter turn after 6 minutes.

> **YIELD: 1 serving**
> **EXCHANGE: 1 bread, 2 high-fat meat**
> **CALORIES: 232**

Ham and Scalloped Potatoes

2	ounces lean ham (diced)	60 g
1	medium potato (peeled and sliced)	1 medium
2	tablespoons onion	30 mL
2	teaspoons parsley	10 mL
	vegetable cooking spray	
¼	cup condensed cream of celery soup	60 mL
¼	cup milk	60 mL
	salt and pepper to taste	

Combine ham, potato, onion, and parsley in baking dish coated with vegetable cooking spray. Blend condensed soup and milk; pour over potato mixture; cover. Bake at 350° F (175° C) for 1 hour, or until potatoes are tender. Add salt and pepper.

MICROWAVE: Cook on High for 10 minutes, or until potatoes are tender. Add salt and pepper.

YIELD: 1 serving
EXCHANGE: 2 lean meat, 1½ bread, ½ milk, ½ fat
CALORIES: 365

Tuna Soufflé

11-ounce can condensed cream of celery soup		300-g can
2	teaspoons parsley (finely chopped)	10 mL
1	teaspoon salt	5 mL
	dash pepper	dash
½	teaspoon marjoram	2 mL
7-ounce can tuna (in water)		200-g can
6	eggs (separated)	6
1	cup mixed vegetables (cooked)	250 mL

Combine condensed soup, parsley, salt, pepper, marjoram, and tuna in saucepan. Heat, stirring constantly, until mixture is hot. Remove from heat and cool slightly. Add egg yolks, one at a time, beating well after each addition. Stir in vegetables. Beat egg whites until soft peaks form. Fold small amount of beaten egg whites into egg yolk mixture, then fold egg yolk mixture into remaining egg whites. Pour into lightly greased 10-inch (25-cm) soufflé dish. Bake at 325° F (165° C) for 50 minutes, or until firm and golden brown. Serve immediately.

YIELD: 8 servings
EXCHANGE 1 SERVING: 1½ lean meat, ⅛ bread, ½ fat
CALORIES 1 SERVING: 134

Hot Tuna Dish

½	cup condensed cream of chicken soup	125 mL
2	ounces chunk tuna (in water)	60 g
2	tablespoons celery (diced)	30 mL
1	tablespoon onion (chopped)	15 mL
1	egg (hard cooked)	1
4	tablespoons potato chips (crushed)	60 mL

Combine condensed soup, tuna, celery, and onion; mix thoroughly. Pour into small casserole. Slice egg; layer egg, then crushed potato chips. Bake at 350° F (175° C) for 20 minutes.

MICROWAVE: Cook on Medium for 7 to 10 minutes.

YIELD: 1 serving
EXCHANGE: 1 ⅓ bread, 3 lean meat, 1 fat
CALORIES: 297

Casserole of Shrimp

2	teaspoons margarine	10 mL
1	tablespoon parsley (chopped)	15 mL
1	tablespoon sherry	15 mL
	dash garlic powder, paprika, cayenne	
½	cup soft bread crumbs	125 mL
3	ounces large shrimp (cooked)	90 g

Melt margarine over low heat. Add parsley, sherry, and seasonings; cook slightly. Add bread crumbs; toss to mix. Place shrimp in small baking dish. Top with bread crumb mixture. Bake at 325° F (165° C) for 20 minutes.

MICROWAVE: Melt margarine; add parsley, sherry, and seasonings. Cook on High for 2 minutes. Add bread crumbs; toss to mix. Place shrimp in small baking dish. Top with bread crumb mixture. Cook on Medium for 5 to 7 minutes.

YIELD: 1 serving
EXCHANGE: 3 high-fat meat, 1 bread
CALORIES: 204

Stuffed Cabbage Rolls

2	large cabbage leaves	2 large
2	ounces ground veal	60 g
2	ounces lean ground beef	60 g
3	tablespoons skim milk	45 mL
1	slice dry bread (crumbled)	1 slice
1	teaspoon onion (grated)	5 mL
	dash salt, pepper, nutmeg	
½	cup beef broth	125 mL
1	tablespoon flour	15 mL

Cook cabbage leaves in boiling salted water until tender; drain. Combine ground veal, beef, skim milk, bread crumbs, onion, salt, pepper, and nutmeg; mix thoroughly. Place half of meat mixture in a cabbage leaf and roll up, tucking ends in. Secure with toothpicks. Place in small baking dish. Repeat with remaining meat mixture and cabbage leaf. Blend beef broth and flour; pour over cabbage rolls. Bake at 350° F (175° C) for 45 to 50 minutes.

MICROWAVE: Cook on Medium for 10 to 12 minutes.

YIELD: 1 serving
EXCHANGE: 4 medium-fat meat, 1 vegetable, 1 bread
CALORIES: 396

Hungarian Goulash

1	tablespoon shortening or margarine	15 mL
1	ounce lean beef (diced)	30 g
1	ounce lean veal (diced)	30 g
1	ounce beef kidney (diced)	30 g
2	teaspoons onion (chopped)	10 mL
1	teaspoon green pepper (chopped)	5 mL
3	cherry tomatoes (halved)	3
½	cup potato (diced)	125 mL
¼	cup carrot (diced)	60 mL
¼	teaspoon salt	1 mL
	dash paprika, pepper, marjoram	

Heat shortening or margarine in skillet; add meat. Brown on all sides; drain. Place in individual casserole. Add remaining ingredients. Add enough water to cover. Cover casserole tightly; bake at 350° F (175° C) for 1 hour.

MICROWAVE: Cook on High for 20 to 25 minutes. Stir halfway through cooking time.

YIELD: 1 serving
EXCHANGE: 3 high-fat meat, 1 bread, 1 vegetable
CALORIES: 348

MEATS AND POULTRY

Steak Roberto

¼	cup margarine	60 mL
1	teaspoon garlic powder	5 mL
1	pound beef tenderloin (8 slices)	500 g
½	teaspoon steak sauce	2 mL
¼	teaspoon bay leaf (crushed)	1 mL
1	tablespoon lemon juice	15 mL
½	teaspoon salt	2 mL
	dash pepper	

Melt margarine and combine with garlic powder. Set aside for 20 minutes to allow flavor to develop. Heat 1 tablespoon (15 mL) of the garlic margarine in heavy skillet until very hot. Place as many beef tenderloin slices as possible in skillet; brown on both sides. Remove to warm steak platter. Repeat with remaining beef, if necessary. Reduce heat. Add remaining garlic margarine to pan. Add steak sauce, bay leaf, lemon juice, salt, and pepper; blend thoroughly. Pour over beef tenderloin on platter.

YIELD: 8 servings
EXCHANGE 1 SERVING: 2 medium-fat meat, ½ fat
CALORIES 1 SERVING: 155

Brisket of Beef with Horseradish

3–4	pound beef brisket	1½–2-kg
1	medium onion (sliced)	1 medium
1	bay leaf	1
1	tablespoon lemon juice	15 mL
½	cup horseradish (grated)	125 mL
	salt and pepper to taste	

Place brisket in large kettle; add salt and pepper. Add onion, bay leaf, and enough water to cover brisket. Bring to a boil. Reduce heat and simmer for 2 hours. Remove brisket from water. Combine lemon juice and horseradish. Rub surface of brisket with horseradish mixture. Return brisket to kettle, cover. Cook 1 hour longer.

EXCHANGE 1 OUNCE (30 G): 1 medium-fat meat
CALORIES 1 OUNCE (30 G): 84

Beef Fondue

1	small tomato	1 small
2	cups beef broth	500 mL
1	bay leaf	1
½	teaspoon rosemary (ground)	2 mL
	sirloin steak (cut into bite-size cubes)	

Peel and crush tomato. Place beef broth, tomato, bay leaf, and rosemary in saucepan; heat to a boil. Pour into fondue pot; keep hot with a burner. Place steak cubes on spear. Cook in hot broth to desired doneness.

EXCHANGE 1 OUNCE (30 G): 1 high-fat meat
CALORIES 1 OUNCE (30 G): 88

Note: Amount of steak used depends on number of servings required.

Sauerbraten

4	ounces lean beef roast	120 g
½	cup beef broth	125 mL
¼	cup water	60 mL
¼	cup cider vinegar	60 mL
¼	teaspoon salt	1 mL
	dash garlic powder	
1	teaspoon margarine	5 mL

Place beef in glass pan or bowl. Combine remaining ingredients, except margarine; pour over beef. Marinate 4 to 5 days in refrigerator. Turn beef at least once a day. Melt margarine in small skillet; add beef and brown. Reduce heat. Add half of the marinade to the skillet. Simmer until beef is tender.

YIELD: 1 serving
EXCHANGE: 4 medium-fat meat
CALORIES: 300

Mushroom-Stuffed Pork Chops

2	tablespoons mushroom pieces	30 mL
1	teaspoon onion (chopped)	5 mL
½	teaspoon parsley (chopped)	2 mL
1	teaspoon raisins (soaked)	5 mL
¼	teaspoon nutmeg	1 mL
1	double pork chop	1

Combine ingredients for stuffing; stir to blend. Split meaty part of chop down to bone; do not split through bone. Fill with stuffing; secure with poultry pins. Place on baking sheet. Bake uncovered at 350° F (175° C) for 35 to 40 minutes, or until tender. Turn once.

YIELD: 1 chop
EXCHANGE 1 OUNCE (30 G): 1 high-fat meat
CALORIES 1 OUNCE (30 G): 109

Teriyaki Pork Steak

	pork steak (thinly sliced)	
½	cup soy sauce	125 mL
1	tablespoon wine vinegar	15 mL
2	tablespoons lemon juice	30 mL
¼	cup water	60 mL
2	tablespoons sugar replacement	30 mL
1½	teaspoons ginger	7 mL
½	teaspoon garlic powder	2 mL

Place slices of pork steak in shallow dish. Combine remaining ingredients; pour over pork. Marinate 1 to 2 hours; turn once. Broil pork 5 to 6 inches (12.5 to 15 cm) from heat, for 2–3 minutes per side. Turn and broil second side.

EXCHANGE 1 OUNCE (30 G): 1 medium-fat meat
CALORIES 1 OUNCE (30 G): 89

Note: Amount of steak used depends on number of servings required.

Calf's Liver

1	tablespoon flour	15 mL
½	teaspoon bay leaf (finely crushed)	2 mL
¼	teaspoon nutmeg	1 mL
	salt and pepper to taste	
½	cup beef broth	125 mL
3	ounces calf's liver	90 g
	vegetable cooking spray	

Combine flour, bay leaf, nutmeg, salt, and pepper in shaker bag. Add liver; shake to coat. Remove liver from bag and shake off excess flour. Brown liver in heavy skillet coated with vegetable cooking spray. Reduce heat. Add beef broth; cover. Simmer for 25 to 30 minutes, or until tender.

YIELD: 1 serving
EXCHANGE: 3 lean meat
CALORIES: 132

Calf's Brains

1	calf's brain (trimmed)	1	
2	tablespoons lemon juice	30 mL	
1	tablespoon cider vinegar	15 mL	
1	teaspoon thyme	5 mL	
1	bay leaf	1	
⅓	cup onion (chopped)	80 mL	
1	parsley sprig (chopped)	1	
⅓	cup celery (chopped)	80 mL	

Rinse brain thoroughly. Cover with water. Add lemon juice and marinate for 2 to 4 hours. Drain. Cover with cold water. Add remaining ingredients. Bring to boil. Cover and simmer for 20 to 25 minutes, or until thoroughly cooked. Remove from heat. Allow to rest 15 minutes. Remove brain from water. Slice thin.

YIELD: 1 brain
EXCHANGE 1 OUNCE (30 G): 1 lean meat
CALORIES 1 OUNCE (30 G): 45

Veal Roast

2–3	pound veal roast	1–1½ kg
2	cups beef broth	500 mL
1	medium onion (sliced)	1 medium
1	bay leaf	1
¼	teaspoon thyme	1 mL
	salt and pepper to taste	

Place roast in heavy kettle or roasting pan. Combine remaining ingredients. Pour over roast. Bake at 375° F (190° C) for 2 to 2½ hours, or until meat is very tender. While baking, baste with pan juices.

EXCHANGE 1 OUNCE (30 G): 1 lean meat
CALORIES 1 OUNCE (30 G): 55

Veal Scaloppine

2	ounces veal steak (boned)	60 g
¼	cup tomato (sieved)	60 mL
2	tablespoons green pepper (chopped)	30 mL
1	tablespoon mushroom pieces	15 mL
1	tablespoon onions (chopped)	15 mL
¼	teaspoon parsley	1 mL
	dash garlic powder, oregano	
	salt and pepper to taste	

Place veal on bottom of individual baking dish. Add remaining ingredients; cover. Bake at 350° F (175° C) for 45 minutes, or until meat is tender.

MICROWAVE: Cook on High for 10 to 12 minutes. Turn and uncover last 2 minutes.

Veal Scaloppine II

½	teaspoon margarine	2 mL
2	ounces veal round steak (thinly sliced)	60 g
2	tablespoons tomato paste	30 mL
6	tablespoons water	90 mL
	dash salt, pepper, oregano, garlic powder	
1	tablespoon mushrooms (sliced)	15 mL
1	teaspoon onion (chopped)	5 mL
1	cup spaghetti (cooked)	250 mL

Melt margarine in small skillet. Brown both sides of slices of veal steak. Place in small baking dish. Blend tomato paste, water, seasonings, mushrooms, and onion together. Pour over veal; cover. Bake at 350° F (175° C) for 30 minutes. Place veal on top of spaghetti. Pour sauce over all.

MICROWAVE: Cook covered on Medium for 12 minutes.

YIELD: 1 serving
EXCHANGE: 2 medium-fat meat, 2 bread
CALORIES: 310

Veal Roll

1	ounce veal (thin slice)	30 g
	salt and pepper to taste	
½	ounce prosciutto (thin slice)	15 g
½	ounce Swiss cheese (thin slice)	15 g
	vegetable cooking spray	

Pound veal slice with mallet or edge of plate until very thin. Add salt and pepper. Place prosciutto on top and roll up. Secure with poultry pin. Brown in heavy skillet coated with vegetable cooking spray. Top with cheese slice. Cover. Cook over low heat just until cheese melts slightly. Serve on hot plate.

YIELD: 1 serving
EXCHANGE: 2 medium-fat meat
CALORIES: 156

Beef Tongue

1	beef tongue

Place tongue in large kettle; cover with water. Add 1 teaspoon (5 mL) salt per quart (L) of water. Bring to boil; reduce heat and simmer 3½ to 4 hours. Remove tongue; immediately place in ice water. Allow to soak 5 minutes. Remove skin and trim. Slice thin. Use for sandwiches.

EXCHANGE 1 OUNCE (30 G): 1 lean meat
CALORIES 1 OUNCE (30 G): 51

Meat Loaf

2	pounds lean ground beef	1 kg
¼	cup onion (grated)	60 mL
1	cup soft bread crumbs	250 mL
1	egg	1
¼	cup parsley (finely snipped)	60 mL
1¼	teaspoons salt	6 mL
	dash pepper, thyme, marjoram	
1	teaspoon evaporated milk	5 mL

Combine all ingredients. Add just enough water to form firm ball. Press into baking dish. Bake at 350° F (175° C) for 1½ hours.

MICROWAVE: Cook on High for 15 minutes. Turn dish halfway through cooking time. Allow to rest for 5 minutes before serving.

YIELD: 12 servings
EXCHANGE 1 SERVING: 2½ lean meat, ¼ bread
CALORIES 1 SERVING: 237

Garlicky Hamburgers

1	pound ground beef	½ kg
½	cup minced onion	125 mL
2	garlic cloves, pressed	2
	Montreal Steak Seasoning	
6	slices cheese	6
1	red onion, sliced thin	1
1	tomato, sliced thin	1
6	large rolls	6
1	head lettuce	1
	sliced pickles	

Mix together ground beef, minced onion, and pressed garlic. Pat into patties and sprinkle with Montreal Steak Seasoning. Grill to your liking. Add cheese until melted. Place hamburger patties on an onion roll and top with a slice of red onion, tomato, lettuce, and pickles.

For a low-carb option, replace the roll with large lettuce leaves wrapped around the burger. If using lettuce, remove the bread exchange from the exchange list.

YIELD: 6 servings
EXCHANGES WITH ROLL: 2½ bread, 2½ meat, 2 fat, 1 vegetable

Klip Klops

4	slices bread (crust removed)	4 slices
½	cup skim milk	125 mL
½	teaspoon garlic powder	2 mL
1	teaspoon onion salt	5 mL
1	pound lean ground beef	500 g
1	egg (beaten)	1
1	quart water	1 L
1	small bay leaf	1 small
1	teaspoon salt	5 mL
1	clove	1

Soak bread in skim milk. Add garlic powder, onion salt, ground beef, and egg; mix thoroughly. Form into 8 balls. Combine water, bay leaf, salt, and clove. Bring to boil. Drop balls into boiling water. Cook until beef is done (about 15 minutes). Drain before placing on hot platter.

YIELD: 8 servings
EXCHANGE 1 SERVING: 2 high-fat meat, 1 bread
CALORIES 1 SERVING: 190

Roast Leg of Lamb

5–6	pound leg of lamb	2½–3 kg
½	cup lo-cal Italian dressing	125 mL
½	cup water	125 mL
3	tablespoons lemon juice	45 mL
1	teaspoon garlic powder	5 mL
½	teaspoon rosemary (ground)	2 mL
½	teaspoon thyme	2 mL
½	teaspoon mace	2 mL
1	teaspoon salt	5 mL
¼	teaspoon pepper	1 mL

Wipe lamb with damp cloth. Puncture lamb with long, sharp spear or poultry pin. Place on a rack in roasting pan, fat side up. Blend remaining ingredients; pour over lamb. Roast uncovered at 325° F (165° C) for 3 to 3½ hours. Baste with pan juices every ½ hour. Add more Italian dressing and water, if necessary.

EXCHANGE 1 OUNCE (30 G): 1 medium-fat meat
CALORIES 1 OUNCE (30 G): 75

Steak Hawaiian

3	ounces beef top round steak (sliced)	90 g
½	teaspoon mace	2 mL
2	tablespoons unsweetened pineapple juice	30 mL
1	pineapple slice (unsweetened)	1

Pound slices of round steak with mallet or edge of plate until thin. Sprinkle both sides with mace. Place in aluminum foil. Sprinkle with pineapple juice; top with pineapple slice. Secure foil tightly. Place in baking dish. Bake at 350° F (175° C) for 40 to 45 minutes.

MICROWAVE: Place in plastic wrap. Cook on High for 10 to 12 minutes.

YIELD: 1 serving
EXCHANGE: 3 lean meat, 1 fruit
CALORIES: 200

Lamb Shish Kebab

4	pounds lean lamb	2 kg
3	garlic cloves (crushed)	3
1½	teaspoons salt	7 mL
1	bay leaf	1
½	teaspoon pepper	2 mL
½	teaspoon ground allspice	2 mL
½	teaspoon ground clove	2 mL
1	teaspoon white vinegar	5 mL
1	cup skim milk	250 mL

Cut lamb into 2-inch (5-cm) cubes. Combine remaining ingredients; blend thoroughly. Pour over lamb in large bowl; cover. Refrigerate overnight. Place lamb pieces on skewers. Barbecue or broil 10 to 15 minutes. Turn once.

EXCHANGE 1 OUNCE (30 G): 1 medium-fat meat
CALORIES 1 OUNCE (3 G): 89

Swiss Steak

1	teaspoon margarine	5 mL
3	ounces beef minute steak	90 g
	salt and pepper to taste	
¼	cup celery (sliced)	60 mL
1	tablespoon onion (chopped)	15 mL
¼	cup tomato (crushed)	60 mL
¼	cup water	60 mL

Heat margarine until very hot. Salt and pepper the steak. Brown both sides; drain. Place in individual baking dish. Add salt, pepper, and remaining ingredients. Cover. Bake at 375° F (190° C) for 1 hour, or until steak is tender.

MICROWAVE: Cook on High 8 to 10 minutes. Uncover last minute.

YIELD: 1 serving
EXCHANGE: 3 medium-fat meat, 1 fat
CALORIES: 220

Roast Duck with Orange Sauce

4–5	pound duck	2–2½ kg
2	medium oranges	2 medium
	salt to taste	
	Orange Sauce (page 148)	

Wash inside and outside of duck thoroughly. Remove any fat from tail or neck opening. Salt interior of bird. Cut each orange (with peel) into 8 sections. Place inside the duck. Secure tail and neck skin, legs, and wings with poultry pins. Salt exterior of duck. Place breast side up on a rack in roasting pan. Bake at 350° F (175° C) for 4 hours. During the final hour, baste with Orange Sauce every 15 minutes.

EXCHANGE 1 OUNCE (30 G): 1 high-fat meat
CALORIES 1 OUNCE (30 G): 96

El Dorado

½	cup chicken broth	125 mL
½	ounce fresh oysters	15 g
1	teaspoon margarine	5 mL
1	tablespoon carrot (grated)	15 mL
2	tablespoons celery (chopped)	30 mL
1	teaspoon parsley (chopped)	5 mL
1	ounce cooked chicken (diced)	30 g
	salt and pepper to taste	

Heat chicken broth to a boil; add oysters. Cook until edges roll; drain. Heat margarine in heavy skillet. Add carrot, celery, and parsley. Sauté until crisp-tender. Add chicken, oysters, and 1 tablespoon (15 mL) of the chicken broth. Cook until thoroughly heated. Drain, if necessary. Add salt and pepper.

YIELD: 1 serving
EXCHANGE: 1 ½ lean meat, 2 fat
CALORIES: 80

Chicken Livers

3	ounces chicken livers	90 g
½	cup skim milk	125 mL
2	tablespoons flour	30 mL
	salt and pepper to taste	
2	teaspoons margarine	10 mL

Soak chicken livers in skim milk overnight. Drain. Combine flour, salt, and pepper in shaker bag. Add livers, one at a time; shake to coat. Remove livers from bag and shake off excess flour. Melt margarine in small skillet; add livers. Cook until lightly browned and tender.

YIELD: 1 serving
EXCHANGE: 3 lean meat, 2 fat
CALORIES: 190

FISH, SEAFOOD, AND EGGS

Fish Florentine

2	tablespoons onion (chopped)	30 mL
½	cup mushrooms (chopped)	125 mL
1	tablespoon margarine	15 mL
2	cups cooked spinach (well drained)	500 mL
1	teaspoon lemon juice	5 mL
1	cup White Sauce (page 147)	250 mL
3	ounces Cheddar cheese (grated)	90 g
12	ounces cooked fish (flaked)	360 g

Sauté onion and mushrooms in margarine until onion is transparent. Add spinach and lemon juice; mix well. Pour into baking dish or 6 individual baking dishes coated with vegetable cooking spray. Cover with ½ cup (125 mL) of the White Sauce. Sprinkle with 1½ ounces (45 mL) of the cheese. Cover with fish, then with remaining sauce. Sprinkle with remaining cheese. Bake at 350° F (175° C) for 20 minutes.

MICROWAVE: Cook on Medium for 10 minutes; turn. Cook 5 minutes more. Hold 3 minutes.

YIELD: 6 servings
EXCHANGE 1 SERVING: 3½ high-fat meat, 1 vegetable, 1 bread, ½ milk, 1 fat
CALORIES 1 SERVING: 215

Note: Yield is not listed for some recipes where some people are allowed 1 exchange while others are allowed 2 or more.

Poached Fish

2	pounds fish (haddock, cod, pollack, salmon)	1 kg
1	quart water	1 L
1	carrot (sliced)	1
1	onion (sliced)	1
1	bay leaf	1
½	teaspoon thyme	2 mL
½	teaspoon whole peppercorns	2 mL

Wash fish; wrap in cheesecloth. Combine remaining ingredients in large kettle. Bring to a boil; reduce heat and cook for 15 minutes. Add fish and cook at a simmer. Time depends on thickness, not weight; cook 10 minutes for each inch (2.5 cm) of thickness. Drain in cheesecloth. Turn out onto warm serving platter. Remove skin carefully.

EXCHANGE 1 OUNCE (30 G): 1 meat
CALORIES 1 OUNCE (30 G): 21

Note: Bone is not counted in serving weight.

Broiled Trout

5	ounce trout fillet	150 g
1	teaspoon margarine	5 mL
	dash lemon, pepper, marjoram, salt, paprika	

Clean trout fillet thoroughly; pat dry. Melt margarine; brush on both sides of fillet. Sprinkle with seasonings in order given. Broil 5 to 6 inches (12.5 to 15 cm) from heat for 10 to 15 minutes. It is not necessary to turn the fillet.

YIELD: 1 serving
EXCHANGE: 5 lean meat, 1 fat
CALORIES: 190

Broiled Smelt

3	ounce smelt	90 g
	salt and pepper to taste	
1	teaspoon margarine	5 mL
1	teaspoon lemon juice	5 mL

Dry smelt thoroughly. Salt and pepper cavity of smelt. Melt margarine; brush on both sides of smelt. Sprinkle with lemon juice. Add salt and pepper. Broil 6 to 8 inches (15 to 20 cm) from heat for 10 to 15 minutes.

YIELD: 1 serving
EXCHANGE: 3 medium-fat meat
CALORIES: 95

Baked White Fish

1	teaspoon margarine	5 mL
3	ounce white fish fillet	90 g
	salt and pepper to taste	

Melt margarine; brush on both sides of fish fillet. Place fish on aluminum foil. Add salt and pepper. Wrap tightly, securing ends. Place on baking sheet. Bake at 375° F (190° C) for 45 minutes.

MICROWAVE: Wrap in plastic wrap; prick wrap. Place on cooking rack. Cook for 7 to 8 minutes, giving package a quarter turn after 4 minutes.

YIELD: 1 serving
EXCHANGE: 3 medium-fat meat, 1 fat
CALORIES: 229

Mustard Halibut Steaks

3	ounce halibut steak	90 g
1	teaspoon margarine	5 mL
1	teaspoon lemon juice	5 mL
½	teaspoon Dijon mustard	2 mL
	dash lemon rind, sugar replacement	
	salt to taste	

Wash and dry halibut thoroughly. Melt margarine; brush on both sides of halibut. Lay on broiler pan. Brush top with mixture of lemon juice, Dijon mustard, and seasonings. Broil 5 to 6 inches (12.5 to 15 cm) from heat for 3 to 4 minutes. Turn halibut; repeat on second side.

YIELD: 1 serving
EXCHANGE: 1 lean meat, 1 fat
CALORIES: 90

Fish Creole

2	pounds white fish fillets	1 kg
3	cups water	750 mL
1	bay leaf	1
3	stalks celery with tops (chopped)	3 stalks
	salt and pepper to taste	
2	cups Creole Sauce (page 140)	500 mL

Cut fish into serving pieces. Combine water, bay leaf, celery, salt, and pepper in saucepan. Boil for 2 to 3 minutes. Remove from heat. Add fish pieces and allow water to cool completely. Drain fish and celery; remove bay leaf. Heat Creole Sauce. Add fish and celery. Simmer on low heat for 5 minutes.

YIELD: 6 servings
EXCHANGE 1 SERVING: 5 medium-fat meat
CALORIES 1 SERVING: 370

Individual Mackerel

3	ounces cooked mackerel (flaked)	90 g
2	tablespoons mushrooms (chopped)	30 mL
1	teaspoon onion (finely chopped)	5 mL
1	teaspoon celery (finely chopped)	5 mL
½	slice bread (crumbled)	½ slice
½	teaspoon parsley (finely chopped)	2 mL
1	egg (beaten)	1
1	teaspoon ketchup	5 mL
	salt and pepper to taste	

Combine all ingredients. Mix thoroughly. Place in small baking dish. Bake at 350° F (175° C) for 40 minutes.

MICROWAVE: Cook on Medium for 10 to 12 minutes.

YIELD: 1 serving
EXCHANGE: 4 medium-fat meat, ½ bread
CALORIES: 322

Baked Turbot

4	ounce turbot fillet	120 g
1	teaspoon margarine	5 mL
1	teaspoon lemon juice	5 mL
	dash salt, pepper, paprika, parsley	

Clean turbot fillet thoroughly; pat dry. Melt margarine; brush on both sides of fillet. Place on aluminum foil. Sprinkle with lemon juice, then seasonings. Wrap up fillet securely; lay in cake pan. Bake at 350° F (175° C) for 30 to 40 minutes. Slide fish out of foil onto warm serving plate.

YIELD: 1 serving
EXCHANGE: 4 medium-fat meat, 1 fat
CALORIES: 400

Salmon Loaf

16	ounces cooked salmon (flaked)	500 g
2	tablespoons onion (chopped)	30 mL
3	tablespoons vegetable juice	45 mL
¼	teaspoon marjoram	1 mL
2	eggs	2
1	cup bread crumbs (finely ground)	250 mL
	salt and pepper to taste	

If canned salmon is used, drain thoroughly. Combine with remaining ingredients. Blend thoroughly. Allow to rest for 5 minutes, or until bread crumbs are soft. Blend again. Line a 9 x 5-inch (23 x 13-cm) loaf pan with waxed paper. Pack salmon mixture tightly into loaf pan. Bake at 350° F (175° C) for 40 minutes.

YIELD: 6 servings
EXCHANGE 1 SERVING: 3 medium-fat meat, ½ bread
CALORIES 1 SERVING: 255

Cooked Flaked Fish

1	pound any raw fish	500 g

Clean fish and cook in salted boiling water for 15 to 20 minutes. Remove skin and bones. Flake fish.

EXCHANGE 1 OUNCE (30 G): 1 meat
CALORIES 1 OUNCE (30 G): 25

Finnan Haddie

3	ounces cooked finnan haddie	90 g
1	tablespoon leek (chopped)	15 mL
1	tablespoon green pepper (chopped)	15 mL
2	teaspoons pimientos (chopped)	10 mL
¼	cup condensed cream of mushroom soup	60 mL
	salt and pepper to taste	
½	ounce Cheddar cheese (grated)	15 g

Arrange finnan haddie in baking dish. Combine leek, green pepper, pimientos, and condensed soup. Stir to mix. Add salt and pepper. Pour over fish. Top with cheese. Bake at 350° F (175° C) for 20 to 25 minutes.

MICROWAVE: Cook on Medium for 10 minutes. Turn once.

YIELD: 1 serving
EXCHANGE: 3½ medium-fat meat
½ bread, 1 fat
CALORIES: 220

Great Crab

1	teaspoon butter	5 mL
	dash lemon juice, parsley, rosemary, salt, paprika	
2	ounces crabmeat	60 g

Melt butter in small saucepan. Mix in lemon juice and seasonings. Add crabmeat. Toss to coat, and heat.

YIELD: 1 serving
EXCHANGE: 2 lean meat, 1 fat
CALORIES: 100

Marinated Crab Legs

½   cup Teriyaki Marinade (page 148) 125 mL
⅓   cup lemon juice   80 mL
½   cup water   125 mL
1   teaspoon basil   5 mL
1–2   pounds cooked crab legs, shelled   500 g–1 kg

Combine marinade, lemon juice, water, and basil. Add crab legs.
(If necessary, add more water to cover legs.) Marinate 2 to 3 hours.

EXCHANGE 1 OUNCE (30 G): 1 lean meat
CALORIES 1 OUNCE (30 G): 32

Oysters on the Shell

2   ounces oysters   60 g
2   tablespoons mushroom pieces   30 mL
1   teaspoon onion (diced)   5 mL
¼   cup vegetable broth   60 mL
1   slice bread (finely crumbled)   1 slice
¼   teaspoon lemon juice   1 mL
      salt and pepper to taste
1   oyster shell   1
¼   ounce Cheddar cheese (grated)   8 g

Cook oysters in small amount of boiling salted water until edges start
to curl. Drain (reserve some liquid). Combine mushrooms, onion, and
broth in saucepan. Bring to a boil. Reduce heat. Add bread crumbs;
stir to mix. Remove from heat. Add lemon juice and enough reserved
oyster liquid to moisten bread-crumb mixture thoroughly. Add oysters,
salt, and pepper. Heap into shell or small baking dish. Top with
cheese. Broil until cheese melts.

YIELD: 1 serving
EXCHANGE: 2½ lean meat, 1 bread
CALORIES: 125

Clam Mousse

1	envelope unflavored gelatin	1 envelope
1	cube vegetable bouillon	1 cube
½	cup boiling water	125 mL
8	ounces minced clams (and juice)	240 g
8	ounces yogurt	240 g
1	teaspoon lemon juice	5 mL
1	teaspoon celery flakes	5 mL
1	teaspoon parsley flakes	5 mL
	small dash cayenne	

Dissolve gelatin and bouillon cube in boiling water. Beat in remaining ingredients with whisk or electric mixer. Pour into mold and chill until firm.

YIELD: 4 servings
EXCHANGE 1 SERVING: 2 lean meat, ¼ milk
CALORIES 1 SERVING: 70

Shrimp Soufflé

2	ounces shrimp (canned)	60 g
	dash thyme, rosemary (crushed), salt, pepper	
1	egg, separated	1
	vegetable cooking spray	

Break shrimp into fine pieces. Add to beaten egg yolk and seasonings. Beat egg white until stiff. Gently stir half of egg white into shrimp mixture. Gently fold in remaining egg white. Pour into large soufflé dish coated with vegetable cooking spray. (Dish should be less than two-thirds full.) Bake at 375° F (190° C) for 15 to 20 minutes.

YIELD: 1 serving
EXCHANGE: 3 lean meat
CALORIES: 205

Tomato Stuffed with Crab Louis

½	teaspoon ketchup	2 mL
1	teaspoon mayonnaise	5 mL
¼	teaspoon Worcestershire sauce	1 mL
1	ounce crabmeat	30 g
1	teaspoon green onion (finely chopped)	5 mL
1	tablespoon celery (finely chopped)	15 mL
1	tablespoon green pepper (finely chopped)	15 mL
1	teaspoon parsley (finely chopped)	5 mL
3	almonds (chopped)	3
1	tomato (peeled)	1
1	lettuce leaf	1

Blend ketchup, mayonnaise, and Worcestershire sauce; add crabmeat, green onion, celery, green pepper, parsley, and almonds. Stir to bind; chill. Cut peeled tomato into 7 sections, slicing almost to the bottom. Fill with Crab Louis. Serve on lettuce leaf.

YIELD: 1 serving
EXCHANGE: 1 medium-fat meat, 1 fat, 1 vegetable
CALORIES: 110

Venetian Seafood

½	cup water	125 mL
2	tablespoons lime juice	30 mL
1	tablespoon chives (finely chopped)	15 mL
1	teaspoon garlic powder	5 mL
½	teaspoon oregano	2 mL
½	teaspoon salt	2 mL
¼	teaspoon pepper	1 mL
1	ounce fresh or frozen lobster (thawed and cubed)	30 g
1	ounce fresh or frozen scallops (thawed)	30 g
1	ounce fresh or frozen shrimp (thawed)	30 g
	vegetable cooking spray	

Make a marinade by blending water, lime juice, and seasonings. Place thawed seafood in deep narrow dish. Pour marinade over seafood to cover. Refrigerate for 3 to 5 hours. (Stir occasionally if seafood is not completely covered with marinade.) Drain. Spray seafood with vegetable cooking spray. Place on baking sheet or dish coated with vegetable cooking spray. Broil 5 to 6 inches (12.5 to 15 cm) from heat for 5–6 minutes until seafood is tender. Shake baking sheet or dish occasionally to brown seafood evenly.

YIELD: 1 serving
EXCHANGE: 3 lean meat
CALORIES: 90

Long Island Boil

1	ounce mussels	30 g
1	tomato (peeled and quartered)	1
1	onion (cut into large chunks)	1
½	teaspoon garlic powder	2 mL
1	teaspoon parsley	5 mL
1	ounce halibut (cut into chunks)	30 g
1	ounce scallops	30 g
	salt and pepper to taste	

Wash mussels thoroughly. Soak in cold water overnight. Steam mussels until shells open; remove mussels from shells. Combine tomato, onion, garlic powder, and parsley. Simmer for 15 minutes. Add halibut and scallops. Cover; simmer 10 minutes. Add mussels, salt, and pepper. Heat thoroughly.

YIELD: 1 serving
EXCHANGE: 3 lean meat, 1 vegetable
CALORIES: 105

Lobster Orientale

1	cup chicken broth	250 mL
4	shallots	4
¼	teaspoon ginger	1 mL
¼	teaspoon curry powder	1 mL
1	ounce pork (cubed)	30 g
2	ounces lobster (cubed)	60 g
1	teaspoon cornstarch	5 mL
¼	cup cold water	60 mL
½	cup bean sprouts	125 mL

Combine chicken broth, shallots, ginger, and curry powder. Heat to a boil. Add pork; cook until tender. Remove from heat. Add lobster. Dissolve cornstarch in cold water. Combine with pork–lobster mixture.

Return to heat; thicken slightly. Add bean sprouts. Heat thoroughly. (Add extra water if mixture thickens too much.)

YIELD: 1 serving
EXCHANGE: 3 medium-fat meat
CALORIES: 140

Shrimp Creole

½	cup Creole Sauce (page 140)	125 mL
10	small shrimp	10
1	cup rice (cooked)	250 mL

Heat Creole Sauce just to a boil. Add shrimp. Remove from heat. Allow to rest 10 minutes. Serve over rice.

YIELD: 1 serving
EXCHANGE: 2 meat, 2 bread, ½ vegetable, 1 fat
CALORIES: 238

Seafood Medley

1	ounce chunk tuna	30 g
1	ounce small shrimp (cooked)	30 g
1	teaspoon lemon juice	5 mL
½	egg (hard cooked and chopped)	½
1	teaspoon green onion (sliced)	5 mL
1	lettuce leaf	1

Combine all ingredients, except lettuce. Chill thoroughly before serving on lettuce leaf with favorite dressing.

YIELD: 1 serving
EXCHANGE: 2½ medium-fat meat, ¼ vegetable
CALORIES: 137

Montana Eggs

1	egg (beaten)	1
½	ounce ham (finely chopped)	15 g
1	teaspoon onion (finely chopped)	5 mL
	salt and pepper to taste	
	vegetable cooking spray	

Combine egg, ham, onion, salt, and pepper in small bowl. Beat to blend. Coat pan with vegetable cooking spray; heat to moderately hot. Add egg mixture. Cook on low heat; stir to scramble.

YIELD: 1 serving
EXCHANGE: 1½ high-fat meat
CALORIES: 125

Basic Omelet

	vegetable cooking spray	
1	egg (well beaten)	1
	salt and pepper to taste	

Coat pan with vegetable cooking spray; heat pan to moderately hot. Add beaten egg and cook over low heat. Lift edges of egg very carefully to allow uncooked portion of egg to run under. Add salt and pepper. When mixture is firm, fold omelet in half, or roll up jelly-roll style. A filling may be added before folding.

YIELD: 1 omelet
EXCHANGE: 1 medium-fat meat
CALORIES: 78

OMELET FILLINGS

Just before folding omelet, add one or more of the following:

Bean Sprouts: ¼ cup (60 mL) bean sprouts

Broccoli: ¼ cup (60 mL) chopped broccoli

Cheese: 1 ounce (30 g) cheese
(EXCHANGE: 1 HIGH-FAT MEAT; CALORIES: 100)

Chicken Liver: 1 ounce (30 g) cooked chopped chicken livers
(EXCHANGE: 1 LEAN MEAT; CALORIES: 45)

Crab: 1 ounce (30 g) flaked crabmeat
(EXCHANGE: 1 LEAN MEAT; CALORIES: 25)

Dried Beef: 1 ounce (30 g) chopped dried beef
(EXCHANGE: 1 MEDIUM-FAT MEAT; CALORIES: 80)

Green Pepper and Celery: 1 tablespoon (15 mL) chopped green pepper, 1 tablespoon (15 mL) chopped celery

Ham: 1 ounce (30 g) ham
(EXCHANGE: 1 HIGH-FAT MEAT; CALORIES: 100)

Herbs: 1 tablespoon (15 mL) chopped parsley,
1 teaspoon (5 mL) chives, dash thyme
(add herbs to beaten egg before cooking)

Mushrooms: 1 tablespoon (15 mL) mushroom pieces

Tomato: 2 tablespoons (30 mL) chopped tomato flesh

Tuna: 1 ounce (30 g) drained water-packed tuna
(EXCHANGE: 1 LEAN MEAT; CALORIES: 50)

Note: Where exchange and calories are listed for filling, these must be added to exchange and calories of omelet.

Eggs Florentine

	vegetable cooking spray	
2	tablespoons cooked spinach (chopped)	30 mL
1	egg	1
	salt and pepper to taste	
½	ounce cheese (grated)	15 g

Spray individual baking dish with vegetable cooking spray. Cover bottom with spinach. Add egg, salt, and pepper. Top with cheese. Bake at 350° F (175° C) for 15 minutes, or until white is set.

MICROWAVE: Prick egg yolk. Cover. Cook on High for 4 to 5 minutes.

YIELD: 1 serving
EXCHANGE: 1 ½ medium-fat meat
CALORIES: 140

Cottage Eggs

3	asparagus spears	3
1	egg	1
	salt and pepper to taste	
1	ounce Swiss cheese (grated)	30 g

Steam asparagus spears until tender. Place in individual baking dish. Poach egg; add salt and pepper. Place on top of asparagus. Top with cheese. Broil until cheese melts.

YIELD: 1 serving
EXCHANGE: 2 high-fat meat, 1 vegetable
CALORIES: 216

Eggs Benedict

half	English muffin	half
1	ounce lean ham slice	30 g
1	egg	1
1	tablespoon Hollandaise Sauce	
	(page 147)	15 mL
	salt and pepper to taste	

Toast muffin half. Cook ham over low heat. Place on muffin. Poach egg and place on top of ham. Spoon Hollandaise Sauce over egg. Add salt and pepper.

YIELD: 1 serving
EXCHANGE: 2⅛ high-fat meat, ½ bread, 1 fat
CALORIES: 266

BREADS

Bran Bread

3	tablespoons shortening	45 mL
3	tablespoons brown sugar replacement	45 mL
3	tablespoons molasses	45 mL
1	teaspoon salt	5 mL
½	cup bran	125 mL
¾	cup boiling water	185 mL
1	package dry yeast	1 package
¼	cup warm water	60 mL
2½	cups flour	625 mL
	margarine (melted)	

Place shortening, brown sugar replacement, molasses, salt, and bran in large mixing bowl. Add boiling water. Stir to blend. Soften dry yeast in warm water. Allow to rest for 5 minutes. Add yeast to bran mixture. Add flour, 1 cup (250 mL) at a time, stirring well between additions, until a soft dough is formed. Knead gently for 10 minutes. Shape into loaf. Place in greased 13 x 9 x 2-inch (33 x 23 x 5-cm) loaf pan. Cover; allow to rise for 2 hours. Punch down; allow to rise for 1 more hour. Bake at 325° F (165° C) for 50 to 55 minutes. Remove to rack and brush lightly with melted margarine.

YIELD: 1 loaf (14 slices)
EXCHANGE 1 SLICE: 1 bread
CALORIES 1 SLICE: 68

Jewish Braid Bread (Challah)

1	package dry yeast	1 package
¾	cup warm water	185 mL
1	teaspoon salt	5 mL
¼	cup sugar replacement	60 mL
2	tablespoons margarine (melted)	30 mL
2	eggs (well beaten)	2
3	cups flour	750 mL
1	teaspoon skim milk	5 mL
	poppy seeds	

Soften yeast in warm water; allow to rest for 55 minutes. Add salt, sugar replacement, and margarine. Measure 1 tablespoon (15 mL) of the beaten eggs. Place in cup and reserve. Add remaining eggs and 1 cup (250 mL) of the flour to yeast mixture; beat vigorously. Add remaining flour. Turn onto floured board and knead until smooth and elastic. Place in lightly greased bowl; cover. Allow to rise until double in size, about 1½ hours. Punch down; divide into thirds. Roll into 3 strips, 18-inches (45-cm) long, with the heel of the hand. Braid the 3 strips loosely, tucking under ends. Blend reserved beaten egg with 1 teaspoon (5 mL) skim milk; carefully brush over braid. Sprinkle with poppy seeds; cover. Allow to rise again until double in size, about 1½ hours. Bake at 350° F (175° C) for 1 hour, or until done.

YIELD: 1 loaf (18 slices)
EXCHANGE 1 SLICE: 1 bread
CALORIES 1 SLICE: 70

Quick Onion Bread

| 1 | loaf frozen bread dough | 1 loaf |
| 1 | package onion soup mix | 1 package |

Allow bread to thaw as directed on package. Roll dough out on unfloured board. Sprinkle half of soup mix over surface. Roll up jelly-roll style. Knead to work mix into dough; repeat with remaining soup mix. Form into loaf. Place in greased 9 x 5-inch (23 x 13-cm) loaf pan; cover. Allow to rise about 2 hours. Bake at 350° F (175° C) for 30 to 40 minutes, or until done.

YIELD: 1 loaf (14 slices)
EXCHANGE 1 SLICE: 1 bread
CALORIES 1 SLICE: 80

Apricot Bread

8	dried apricot halves	8
1/3	cup shortening	80 mL
1/4	cup (packed) brown sugar replacement	60 mL (packed)
2	eggs (beaten)	2
1	cup skim milk	250 mL
1/2	teaspoon salt	2 mL
1 1/2	teaspoons baking powder	7 mL
1/4	teaspoon cinnamon	1 mL
	dash nutmeg	
3/4	cup flour	185 mL

Soak apricots in warm water for 2 hours. Cook over medium heat for 10 minutes; drain and chop fine. Cream shortening and brown sugar replacement. Add eggs and skim milk; beat thoroughly. Add salt, baking powder, cinnamon, and nutmeg. Stir in apricots and enough of the flour to make a thick cake batter. Pour into greased 9 x 5-inch (23 x 13-cm) loaf pan. Bake at 350° F (175° C) for 1 1/2 hours, or until toothpick comes out clean.

MICROWAVE: Bake on Low for 20 minutes. Increase heat to High for 5 minutes, or until toothpick comes out clean. Hold 2 minutes. Turn pan a quarter turn every 10 minutes.

YIELD: 1 loaf (14 slices)
EXCHANGE 1 SLICE: 1 bread, 1 fat
CALORIES: 75

Raisin Bread

1	package dry yeast	1 package
¼	cup warm water	60 mL
¾	cups milk (scalded and cooled)	185 mL
2	tablespoons sugar replacement	30 mL
1	teaspoon salt	5 mL
1	egg	1
2	tablespoons margarine (softened)	30 mL
3¾	cups flour	940 mL
1	cup raisins	250 mL

Soften yeast in warm water; allow to rest for 5 minutes. Combine milk, sugar replacement, salt, egg, and margarine; mix thoroughly. Stir in yeast mixture. Add 1 cup (250 mL) of the flour. Beat until smooth. Mix in raisins. Blend in remaining flour. Knead for 5 minutes. Cover; allow to rise for 2 hours. Punch down; form into loaf. Place in greased 9 x 5-inch (23 x 13-cm) loaf pan; cover. Allow to rise for 1 hour. Bake at 400° F (200° C) for 30 minutes, or until loaf sounds hollow and is golden brown. Remove to rack.

YIELD: 1 loaf (14 slices)
EXCHANGE 1 SLICE: 1 bread
CALORIES 1 SLICE: 68

Pita Bread

1	package dry yeast	1 package
½	teaspoon sugar replacement	2 mL
1	teaspoon salt	5 mL
1	tablespoon liquid shortening	15 mL
1½	cups warm water	375 mL
4	cups flour	1,000 mL

Dissolve yeast, sugar, salt, and liquid shortening in warm water. Add 3 cups (750 mL) of the flour; stir to mix well. (Dough should be fairly stiff; if not, add more flour.) Turn out onto floured surface; knead in remaining flour. (Dough will be very stiff.) Form into 15½-inch (39-cm) tube. Cut into 15 slices. Pat to make circles about 6 inches (15 cm) in diameter. Lay on lightly greased baking pans; cover. Allow to rise until almost doubled, about 1½–2 hours. Bake at 475° F (245° C) for 10 to 12 minutes, or until lightly golden brown, puffed, and hollow. These freeze well.

YIELD: 15 pita bread pockets
EXCHANGE 1 POCKET: 1½ bread, ½ fat
CALORIES 1 POCKET: 70

Pioneer Cornbread

1	egg	1
1	cup skim milk	250 mL
2	tablespoons lo-cal maple syrup	30 mL
2	tablespoons margarine (melted)	30 mL
⅔	cup cornmeal	160 mL
¾	cup flour	185 mL
1	tablespoon baking powder	15 mL
1	teaspoon salt	5 mL

Beat egg until light and lemon colored. Add skim milk, maple syrup, and margarine. Combine cornmeal, flour, baking powder, and salt in large bowl. Stir to blend. Gradually add flour mixture to liquid. Pour into greased 8-inch (20-cm) square pan. Bake at 425° F (220° C) for 20 to 25 minutes.

MICROWAVE: Bake on Low for 10 minutes. Increase heat to High for 5 minutes, or until toothpick comes out clean.

YIELD: 9 squares
EXCHANGE 1 SQUARE: 1½ bread
CALORIES 1 SQUARE: 82

Baking Powder Biscuits

1	cup flour	250 mL
1	teaspoon baking powder	5 mL
¼	teaspoon yeast	1 mL
¼	teaspoon salt	1 mL
1	tablespoon liquid shortening	15 mL
6	tablespoons milk	90 mL
	vegetable cooking spray	

Combine all ingredients, except vegetable cooking spray; mix just until blended. Turn out on floured board. Roll out to a ½-inch (1-cm) thickness. Cut into circles with floured 2-inch (5-cm) cutter. Place on baking sheet coated with vegetable cooking spray; cover. Allow to rest for 10 minutes. Bake at 450° F (230° C) for 12 to 15 minutes, or until lightly browned.

YIELD: 10 biscuits
EXCHANGE 1 BISCUIT: 1 bread, ½ fat
CALORIES 1 BISCUIT: 90

Yeast Rolls

1	package dry yeast	1 package
¼	cup warm water	60 mL
2	tablespoons sugar replacement	30 mL
2	teaspoons salt	10 mL
1	tablespoon margarine (melted)	15 mL
¾	cup warm water	185 mL
3½	cups flour	875 mL
1	egg (well beaten)	1

Soften yeast in the ¼ cup (60 mL) warm water. Allow to rest for 5 minutes. Combine sugar replacement, salt, margarine, and the ¾ cup (185 mL) warm water; stir to mix. Add 1 cup (250 mL) of the flour; beat well. Blend in yeast mixture and the egg. Add remaining flour; mix well. Knead gently until dough is smooth; cover. Allow to rise for 1 hour. Punch down. Allow to rise for 1 more hour. Punch down. Allow to rest for 10 minutes. Shape into 36 rolls. Place on greased cookie sheet or in greased muffin tins. Allow to rise until doubled in size, about 1½–2 hours. Bake at 400° F (200° C) for 20 to 25 minutes, or until golden brown.

YIELD: 36 rolls
EXCHANGE 1 ROLL: 1 bread
CALORIES 1 ROLL: 68

Orange Muffins

1	cup orange juice	250 mL
1	tablespoon orange peel (grated)	15 mL
½	cup raisins (soaked)	125 mL
⅓	cup sugar replacement	80 mL
1	tablespoon margarine	15 mL
1	egg	1
¼	teaspoon salt	1 mL
1	teaspoon baking soda	5 mL

1	teaspoon baking powder	5 mL
½	teaspoon vanilla extract	2 mL
2	cups flour	500 mL

Combine orange juice, orange peel, and raisins. Allow to rest for 1 hour. Cream together the sugar replacement, margarine, and egg. Add salt, baking soda, baking powder, and vanilla extract. Stir in orange juice mixture. Stir in enough of the flour to make a thick cake batter. Spoon into greased muffin tins, filling no more than two-thirds full. Bake at 350° F (175° C) for 20 to 25 minutes, or until done.

MICROWAVE: Spoon into 6-ounce (180-mL) custard cups, filling no more than two-thirds full. Cook on Low for 7 to 8 minutes. Increase heat to High for 2 minutes, or until done.

YIELD: 24 muffins
EXCHANGE 1 MUFFIN: 1 bread
CALORIES 1 MUFFIN: 68

Fresh Apple Muffins

2	tablespoons soft margarine	30 mL
2	tablespoons sugar replacement	30 mL
1	egg (beaten)	1
1¼	cups flour	310 mL
¼	teaspoon salt	1 mL
2	teaspoons baking powder	10 mL
6	tablespoons skim milk	90 mL
1	small apple (peeled and chopped)	1 small

Cream margarine and sugar replacement; add egg. Stir in remaining ingredients. Spoon into greased muffin tins, filling no more than two-thirds full. Bake at 400° F (200° C) for 25 minutes, or until done.

YIELD: 12 muffins
EXCHANGE 1 MUFFIN: 1 bread
CALORIES 1 MUFFIN: 72

Popovers

1	cup flour	250 mL
½	teaspoon salt	2 mL
2	eggs	2
1	cup skim milk	250 mL

Sift flour and salt together; set aside. Beat eggs and skim milk; add to flour. Beat until smooth and creamy. Pour into heated greased muffin tins, filling half full or less. Bake at 375° F (190° C) for 50 minutes, or until popovers are golden brown and sound hollow. Do not open oven for first 40 minutes.

> **YIELD: 18 popovers**
> **EXCHANGE 1 POPOVER: ½ bread, ⅛ meat**
> **CALORIES 1 POPOVER: 44**

Soya Crisps

1	cup soy flour	250 mL
1	cup chicken broth	250 mL
1	tablespoon liquid shortening	15 mL
1	teaspoon salt	5 mL

Blend soy flour and broth in saucepan until smooth. Bring gradually to a boil; remove from heat. Blend in liquid shortening and salt. Pour into large flat baking sheet to a depth of no more than ¼ inch (6 mm). Bake at 325° F (165° C) for 30 minutes. Cool slightly. Cut into 2¼-inch (5.5-cm) squares. Cut diagonally into triangles.

> **YIELD: 80 crisps**
> **EXCHANGE 10 CRISPS: 1 lean meat**
> **CALORIES 10 CRISPS: 50**

Cake Doughnuts

1	tablespoon granulated sugar	15 mL
4	tablespoons sugar replacement	60 mL
⅓	cup buttermilk	80 mL
1	egg (well beaten)	1
1	cup flour	250 mL
⅛	teaspoon baking soda	½ mL
1	teaspoon baking powder	5 mL
	dash nutmeg, cinnamon, vanilla extract, salt	
	oil for deep-fat frying	

Combine sugars, buttermilk, and egg; beat well. Add remaining ingredients, except oil. Beat just until blended. Heat oil to 375° F (190° C). Drop dough from doughnut dropper into hot fat. Fry until golden brown, turning often. Drain.

YIELD: 12 doughnuts
EXCHANGE 1 DOUGHNUT: 1 bread, 1 fat
CALORIES 1 DOUGHNUT: 130

Tea Scones

1	cup flour	250 mL
1	teaspoon baking powder	5 mL
¼	teaspoon salt	1 mL
1	tablespoon sugar replacement	15 mL
¼	cup margarine (cold)	60 mL
1	egg	1
¼	cup evaporated (skim) milk	60 mL

Sift flour, baking powder, salt, and sugar replacement. Cut in cold margarine as for pie crust. Beat egg and evaporated milk together thoroughly; stir into flour mixture. Knead gently on lightly floured board. Divide dough in half; roll each half into a circle. Cut circles into quarters. Place on lightly greased cookie sheet. Brush tops with milk. Bake at 450° F (230° C) for 15 minutes, or until done.

YIELD: 8 scones
EXCHANGE 1 SCONE: 1 bread
CALORIES 1 SCONE: 34

Scone Variations

APPLE

8 chopped, dried apple halves
EXCHANGE 1 SCONE: 1 bread, ¼ fruit
CALORIES 1 SCONE: 44

APRICOT

8 chopped, dried apricot halves
EXCHANGE 1 SCONE: 1 bread, ¼ fruit
CALORIES 1 SCONE: 44

CRANBERRY

¼ cup (60 mL) chopped cranberries
EXCHANGE 1 SCONE: 1 bread
CALORIES 1 SCONE: 34

DATES

8 chopped dates
EXCHANGE 1 SCONE: 1 bread, ½ fruit
CALORIES 1 SCONE: 54

LEMON

1 tablespoon (15 mL) grated lemon peel
EXCHANGE 1 SCONE: 1 bread
CALORIES 1 SCONE: 34

ORANGE

1½ tablespoons (25 mL) grated orange peel
EXCHANGE 1 SCONE: 1 bread
CALORIES 1 SCONE: 34

PEACHES

8 chopped dried peach halves
EXCHANGE 1 SCONE: 1 bread, ½ fruit
CALORIES 1 SCONE: 54

RAISIN

4 tablespoons (60 mL) raisins
EXCHANGE 1 SCONE: 1 bread, ¼ fruit
CALORIES 1 SCONE: 44

Potato Dumplings

1	small cooked potato	1 small
1	egg (beaten)	1
2	tablespoons flour	30 mL
	salt and pepper to taste	

With a fork, break up and mash the potato. Combine with the remaining ingredients. Beat until light and fluffy. Drop by tablespoonfuls on top of boiling salted water or beef broth. Boil for 5 minutes, or until dumplings rise to surface. Good with Sauerbraten (page 59).

YIELD: 3 or 4 dumplings
EXCHANGE: 1 bread, 1 meat
CALORIES: 140

Baked Sweet Potato

¼	cup sweet potato or yam (mashed)	60 mL
	dash salt, pepper, nutmeg	
1	tablespoon milk	15 mL

Combine all ingredients. Beat until smooth and creamy. Bake at 350° F (175° C) for 20 minutes.

YIELD: 1 serving
EXCHANGE: 1 bread
CALORIES: 75

Mountain Man Pancakes

1	egg	1
1¼	cups buttermilk	310 mL
1	tablespoon molasses	15 mL
2	tablespoons margarine (melted)	30 mL
1	cup flour	250 mL
1	teaspoon salt	5 mL
½	teaspoon baking soda	2 mL
½	teaspoon baking powder	2 mL
½	cup yellow cornmeal	125 mL
	vegetable cooking spray	

Beat egg, buttermilk, molasses, and margarine together until well blended. Add remaining ingredients, except vegetable cooking spray. Stir just enough to blend. Cook in skillet coated with vegetable cooking spray.

YIELD: 10 pancakes, 4 inches (10 cm) in diameter each
EXCHANGE 1 PANCAKE: 1 bread, 1 fat
CALORIES 1 PANCAKE: 95

Potato Pancake

1	medium raw potato (grated)	1 medium
1	egg	1
2	tablespoons flour	30 mL
2	teaspoons salt	10 mL
2	teaspoons chives	10 mL
	vegetable cooking spray	

Place grated potato in ice water. Allow to stand for 30 minutes to an hour. Drain; pat potato dry. Place potato in bowl; add egg, flour, salt, and chives. Stir to blend. Divide mixture into 4 parts and spoon into large skillet coated with vegetable cooking spray. Brown on both sides.

YIELD: 4 pancakes
EXCHANGE 2 PANCAKES: 1 bread, ½ medium-fat meat
CALORIES 2 PANCAKES: 80

Potato Puffs

½	cup potatoes (cooked and mashed or whipped)	125 mL
1	cup flour	250 mL
1½	teaspoons baking powder	7 mL
½	teaspoon salt	2 mL
1	egg (well beaten)	1
½	cup milk	125 mL
	oil for deep-fat frying	

With a fork, break up and mash enough potatoes to fill a small cup. Combine with remaining ingredients, except oil. Beat well. Heat oil to 375° F (190° C). From tablespoon, drop a walnut-size piece of dough into hot fat. Remove when puff rises to the surface (about 2–3 minutes) and is golden brown. Repeat with remaining dough. Drain.

Cornbread Stuffing

6	tablespoons butter	90 mL
1	large onion (chopped)	1 large
1	cup celery with tops (chopped)	250 mL
1	teaspoon thyme	5 mL
1	teaspoon sage	5 mL
1	tablespoon salt	15 mL
1	teaspoon pepper	5 mL
6	cups cornbread crumbs	1.5 L

Melt butter in medium saucepan. Add onion, celery, thyme, sage, salt, and pepper. Sauté over low heat for 3 to 4 minutes. Remove from heat. Add cornbread crumbs; toss to mix. Add water to moisten stuffing consistency.

YIELD: 6 cups (1.5 L)
EXCHANGE ½ CUP (125 mL): 1 bread, 1 fat
CALORIES ½ CUP (125 mL): 125

Prune–Apple Stuffing

1	cup prunes (soaked and chopped)	250 mL
1½	cups apples (chopped)	375 mL
½	cup raisins	125 mL
1	teaspoon cinnamon	5 mL
½	teaspoon nutmeg	2 mL

Combine fruit and spices; mix thoroughly. Allow to rest for 10 minutes before using.

YIELD: 3 cups (750 mL)
EXCHANGE ¼ CUP (60 mL): 1 fruit
CALORIES ¼ CUP (60 mL): 60

Herb-Seasoned Stuffing

1	pound loaf bread (2–3 days old)	500-g loaf
½	cup butter or margarine	125 mL
1	teaspoon thyme	5 mL
1	teaspoon sage	5 mL
1	teaspoon rosemary	5 mL
1	teaspoon dried lemon rind	5 mL

Remove crust from bread; cut bread into cubes. Melt butter or margarine in large skillet. Add seasonings; stir to mix. Add bread cubes. Toss or stir lightly to coat bread cubes. Pour onto baking sheet. Allow to dry by air or dry in very slow oven. (These dried bread cubes are good as croutons.) Add salt and water to moisten when ready to use as stuffing.

YIELD: 8 cups (2 L)
EXCHANGE ½ CUP (125 mL): 1 bread, 1 fat
CALORIES ½ CUP (125 mL): 75

Baked Rice

1	cube beef bouillon	1 cube
1	cup hot water	250 mL
¼	cup rice	60 mL
1	green onion (chopped)	1
2	tablespoons celery (chopped)	30 mL
3	tablespoons dry bread crumbs	45 mL

Dissolve bouillon in hot water. Add rice, green onion, and celery; cover. Cook for 5 minutes. Add bread crumbs. Pour into small baking dish. Bake at 350° F (175° C) for 25 to 30 minutes, or until top is lightly crusted.

YIELD: 1 serving
EXCHANGE: 1½ bread
CALORIES: 115

Rice Pilaf

½	cup rice	125 mL
1	teaspoon butter	5 mL
½	teaspoon salt	2 mL
1	tablespoon lemon juice	15 mL
1	cup boiling water	250 mL

Sauté rice in butter over low heat in large saucepan. Add remaining ingredients. Bring to a boil. Reduce heat; cover. Simmer until water is absorbed. Fluff with fork before serving.

YIELD: 1 cup (250 mL)
EXCHANGE: 2 bread, 1 fat
CALORIES: 150

Corn Pudding

16-ounce can corn		500-g can
1	egg (beaten)	1
1	teaspoon pimiento (chopped)	5 mL
1	teaspoon green pepper	5 mL
1	teaspoon margarine (melted)	5 mL
1	teaspoon sugar replacement	5 mL
¾	cup milk	185 mL
	salt and pepper to taste	
	vegetable cooking spray	

Combine all ingredients, except vegetable cooking spray. Pour into baking dish coated with vegetable cooking spray. Bake at 325° F (165° C) for 35 to 40 minutes, or until firm.

YIELD: 6 servings
EXCHANGE 1 SERVING: 1 bread, 1 fat
CALORIES 1 SERVING: 55

VEGETABLES

ABC's of Vegetables

1	cup asparagus pieces	250 mL
1	cup broccoli florets	250 mL
1	cup carrot slices	250 mL
1	cup spinach (chopped)	250 mL
	vegetable cooking spray	
	11-ounce can condensed cream of mushroom soup	300-g can
2	tablespoons onions (finely chopped)	30 mL
1	teaspoon thyme	5 mL
½	cup water	125 mL
	salt and pepper to taste	

Layer asparagus, broccoli, carrots, and spinach in a baking dish coated with vegetable cooking spray. Blend remaining ingredients. Pour over vegetables. Cover. Bake at 350° F (175° C) for 30 to 40 minutes, or until vegetables are tender.

YIELD: 8 servings
EXCHANGE 1 SERVING: 1 vegetable, ½ bread, ½ fat
CALORIES 1 SERVING: 42

Baked Eggplant

1	slice eggplant	1 slice
1	slice onion	1 slice
1	ounce sharp Cheddar cheese (shredded)	30 g
2	tablespoons condensed tomato soup	30 mL
1	teaspoon dry bread crumbs	5 mL
¼	teaspoon thyme	1 mL
¼	teaspoon salt	1 mL
	dash pepper	

Cook eggplant and onion in small amount of water until tender. Drain; reserve liquid. Place eggplant and onion in small baking dish. Top with cheese. Blend condensed soup, 1 tablespoon (15 mL) of the eggplant liquid, bread crumbs, thyme, salt, and pepper. Pour over eggplant; cover. Bake at 350° F (175° C) for 30 minutes.

MICROWAVE: Uncover. Cook on High for 5 minutes. Turn after 2 minutes.

YIELD: 1 serving
EXCHANGE: 1 high-fat meat, 1 vegetable
CALORIES: 161

Cheese Tomato

1	tomato (thickly sliced)	1
	vegetable cooking spray	
	dash celery salt, garlic salt, pepper	
1	ounce American cheese (grated)	30 g

Place tomato slices on broiler pan coated with vegetable cooking spray. Sprinkle with seasonings. Top with cheese. Broil 5 to 6 inches (12.5 to 15 cm) from heat until cheese is melted.

YIELD: 1 serving
EXCHANGE: 1 vegetable, 1 high-fat meat
CALORIES: 140

Okra and Tomatoes

2	cups okra	500 mL
¼	cup vinegar	60 mL
2	cups tomatoes (cut into eighths)	500 mL
1	cup onions (coarsely chopped)	250 mL
½	cup green pepper (coarsely chopped)	125 mL
	sprig parsley (chopped)	
1	tablespoon mint (chopped)	15 mL
1	teaspoon garlic powder	5 mL
	salt and pepper to taste	
	vegetable cooking spray	

Soak okra in vinegar for 5 minutes. Drain. Pat okra slightly dry. Combine all ingredients (except vinegar) in baking dish coated with vegetable cooking spray. Cover. Bake at 350° F (175° C) for 45 minutes.

YIELD: 5 servings
EXCHANGE 1 SERVING: 1 vegetable
CALORIES 1 SERVING: 31

Kohlrabi

2	cups kohlrabi (cut into strips)	500 mL
2	teaspoons butter	10 mL
2	tablespoons fresh parsley (chopped)	30 mL
	salt and pepper to taste	

Cook kohlrabi in boiling salted water until soft; drain. Melt butter (or margarine) in saucepan. Add parsley; sauté over low heat for 2 minutes. Add kohlrabi. Toss to coat. Add salt and pepper.

YIELD: 4 servings
EXCHANGE 1 SERVING: 1 vegetable, ½ fat
CALORIES 1 SERVING: 36

Italian Asparagus

½	pound asparagus spears (cooked or canned)	250 g
	vegetable cooking spray	
¼	cup Tomato Sauce (page 140)	60 mL
¼	cup water	60 mL
½	teaspoon oregano	2 mL
¼	teaspoon garlic powder	1 mL
	salt and pepper to taste	
¼	cup Swiss cheese (grated)	60 mL

Lay asparagus spears in shallow baking dish coated with vegetable cooking spray. Blend Tomato Sauce, water, oregano, garlic powder, salt, and pepper. Spread evenly over spears. Top with grated cheese. Bake at 350° F (175° C) for 20 to 25 minutes.

MICROWAVE: Cook on High for 5 to 6 minutes.

YIELD: 4 servings
EXCHANGE 1 SERVING: ½ vegetable, ½ medium-fat meat
CALORIES 1 SERVING: 58

Cauliflower au Gratin

2	cups cauliflowerets	500 mL
1	teaspoon salt	5 mL
1	teaspoon butter	5 mL
1	teaspoon flour	5 mL
1	cup milk (cold)	250 mL
¼	cup American cheese (diced)	60 mL
	vegetable cooking spray	
	salt and pepper to taste	

Place cauliflowerets in large kettle. Fill with enough water to cover. Add salt. Bring to a boil; cook 5 minutes. Drain; rinse with cold water. Melt butter (or margarine) in saucepan. Blend flour with cold milk. Add to melted butter. Cook over low heat, stirring constantly, until slightly thickened. Add cheese; cook until cheese is completely blended. Place cauliflower in baking dish coated with vegetable cooking spray; add salt and pepper. Cover with cheese topping. Bake at 350° F (175° C) for 20 minutes.

YIELD: 4 servings
EXCHANGE 1 SERVING: 1 vegetable, ½ medium-fat meat
CALORIES 1 SERVING: 119

Brussels Sprouts and Mushrooms au Gratin

1	tablespoon butter	15 mL
2	cups Brussels sprouts	500 mL
1	cup mushroom pieces	250 mL
	salt and pepper to taste	
2	ounces Swiss cheese (grated)	60 g

Melt butter in skillet. Lightly sauté Brussels sprouts and mushrooms. Add salt and pepper. Remove from heat and pour into baking dish. Cover with cheese. Bake at 350° F (175° C) for 20 to 25 minutes.

MICROWAVE: Cook on Medium for 10 minutes. Turn once.

YIELD: 4 servings
EXCHANGE 1 SERVING: 1 high-fat meat, ½ vegetable
CALORIES 1 SERVING: 65

Baked Vegetable Medley

1	cup 2-inch (5-cm) cubes eggplant	250 mL
1	cup 2-inch (5-cm) slices okra	250 mL
1	cup bean sprouts	250 mL
½	cup small mushrooms	125 mL
1	onion (cut into eighths)	1
	vegetable cooking spray	
11-ounce	can condensed cream of celery soup	300-g can
¼	cup water	60 mL
	salt and pepper to taste	
1	slice bread (finely crumbled)	1 slice

Combine all vegetables in baking dish coated with vegetable cooking spray. Blend condensed soup and water; add salt and pepper. Pour over vegetables. Top with bread crumbs. Cook at 325° F (165° C) for 25 to 30 minutes, or until hot, and crumbs are golden brown.

YIELD: 8 servings
EXCHANGE 1 SERVING: 1 vegetable, ½ bread
CALORIES 1 SERVING: 49

Shredded Cabbage

1	head cabbage (coarsely shredded)	1 head
2	teaspoons butter	10 mL
½	teaspoon nutmeg	2 mL
	salt and pepper to taste	

Cook cabbage in a small amount of boiling salted water until tender; drain. Press out excess moisture or pat dry. Melt butter in skillet. Add nutmeg; stir to blend. Add cabbage; toss to coat. Add salt and pepper.

YIELD: 4 servings
EXCHANGE 1 SERVING: ½ vegetable, ½ fat
CALORIES 1 SERVING: 32

Irish Vegetables

1	bay leaf	1
1	cup water	250 mL
2	tablespoons wine vinegar	30 mL
½	cup corn	125 mL
½	cup celery (sliced)	125 mL
½	cup broccoli florets	125 mL
½	cup carrot (sliced)	125 mL
½	cup cauliflowerets	125 mL
¼	cup pimiento (chopped)	60 mL
	salt and pepper to taste	

Combine bay leaf, water, and wine vinegar in medium saucepan.
Bring to a boil; add vegetables. Simmer until vegetables are tender.
Drain; remove bay leaf. Add salt and pepper.

YIELD: 5 servings
EXCHANGE 1 SERVING: 1 vegetable
CALORIES 1 SERVING: 51

Spiced Bean Sprouts

2	cups bean sprouts	500 mL
½	teaspoon caraway seeds	2 mL
½	teaspoon basil	2 mL
2	teaspoons butter	10 mL
	salt and pepper to taste	

Combine bean sprouts, caraway seeds, and basil in saucepan with
small amount of water. Cook until hot and tender; drain. Place in
serving dish; top with butter, salt, and pepper. Toss to coat.

YIELD: 4 servings
EXCHANGE 1 SERVING: ½ vegetable, ½ fat
CALORIES 1 SERVING: 25

German Green Beans

2	cups green beans	500 mL
1	slice bacon	1 slice
¼	cup onion (chopped)	60 mL
1	teaspoon flour	5 mL
¼	cup vinegar	60 mL
½	cup water	125 mL
2	tablespoons sugar replacement	30 mL

Cook green beans in boiling salted water until tender; drain. Cut bacon into ½-inch (12-mm) pieces. Place in skillet; add onion. Sauté until bacon is crisp and onion is tender; drain. Blend flour, vinegar, water, and sugar replacement in screw-top jar. Pour over bacon and onion. Cook over low heat to thicken slightly. Add green beans.

YIELD: 4 servings
EXCHANGE 1 SERVING: ½ vegetable, ¼ bread, ½ fat
CALORIES 1 SERVING: 52

Pizza Beans

2	cups green beans	500 mL
1	tablespoon lemon juice	15 mL
¼	teaspoon oregano	1 mL
1	teaspoon pimiento (chopped)	5 mL
	dash garlic powder, salt	

Cook green beans in boiling salted water until tender; drain. Combine lemon juice, oregano, pimiento, garlic powder, and salt. Pour over beans; toss.

YIELD: 5 servings
EXCHANGE 1 SERVING: ½ vegetable
CALORIES 1 SERVING: 32

Whipped Summer Squash

3	cups summer squash	750 mL
¼	cup evaporated milk	60 mL
2	teaspoons butter	10 mL
	salt and pepper to taste	

Peel and cut squash into small pieces. Place in saucepan with small amount of water. Bring to a boil; reduce heat and simmer until squash is crisp-tender. Drain. Beat squash with rotary beater; add evaporated milk and butter. Beat until light and fluffy. Add salt and pepper.

YIELD: 4 servings
EXCHANGE 1 SERVING: 1 vegetable, 1 fat
CALORIES 1 SERVING: 68

Spiced Beets

½	cup wine vinegar	125 mL
¼	cup water	60 mL
1	bay leaf	1
1	whole clove	1
1	teaspoon black pepper	5 mL
3	tablespoons sugar replacement	45 mL
2	cups beets (sliced)	500 mL

Combine all ingredients except beets. Bring to a boil. Add beets; simmer for 10 minutes, or until tender.

MICROWAVE: Combine all ingredients, except beets. Cook on High for 2 minutes. Add beets. Cook on Medium for 2 minutes.

YIELD: 4 servings
EXCHANGE 1 SERVING: 1 vegetable
CALORIES 1 SERVING: 36

Indian Squash

2	cups acorn squash (cubed)	500 mL
2	teaspoons margarine	10 mL
1	teaspoon orange rind	5 mL
¼	cup orange juice	60 mL
2	tablespoons sugar replacement	30 mL

Cook squash in small amount of boiling water until crisp-tender; drain. Melt margarine in saucepan. Add orange rind, juice, and sugar replacement. Cook over low heat until sugar is dissolved. Add squash; cover. Continue cooking until squash is tender.

YIELD: 4 servings
EXCHANGE 1 SERVING: 1 bread, ½ fat
CALORIES 1 SERVING: 60

Beans Orientale

1½	cups French-cut green beans (cooked)	375 mL
2	tablespoons almonds (blanched and slivered)	30 mL
½	cup mushroom pieces	125 mL
2	teaspoons butter	10 mL
	salt and pepper to taste	

Heat green beans; drain. Sauté almonds and mushrooms in butter. Add green beans. Add salt and pepper.

MICROWAVE: Melt butter in bowl. Add almonds and mushrooms. Cover. Cook on High for 30 seconds. Add green beans. Cook on Medium for 2 to 3 minutes.

YIELD: 4 servings
EXCHANGE 1 SERVING: ½ vegetable, ½ fat
CALORIES 1 SERVING: 45

Vegetable Casserole

1	cup peas	250 mL
1	cup green beans	250 mL
1	cup carrots (sliced)	250 mL
1	cup mushrooms	250 mL
1	egg	1
1	teaspoon margarine (melted)	5 mL
½	cup milk	125 mL
	salt and pepper to taste	
	vegetable cooking spray	

Cook vegetables in small amount of boiling salted water until crisp-tender; drain. Chop vegetables fine. Whip egg until lemon colored; add margarine and milk. Blend well. Add chopped vegetables, salt, and pepper. Pour into baking dish coated with vegetable cooking spray. Cover. Bake at 350° F (175° C) for 45 minutes, or until set.

YIELD: 8 servings
EXCHANGE 1 SERVING: 1 vegetable
CALORIES 1 SERVING: 36

Pea Pod–Carrot Sauté

1	cup pea pods	250 mL
1	cup carrots (sliced)	250 mL
1	teaspoon salt	5 mL
2	teaspoons margarine	10 mL
1	tablespoon Worcestershire sauce	15 mL

Combine pea pods and carrots in saucepan. Cover with water; add salt. Cook until tender; drain. Melt margarine in saucepan. Add Worcestershire sauce; stir to blend. Add pea pods and carrots. Toss to coat.

YIELD: 4 servings
EXCHANGE 1 SERVING: ½ bread, ½ fat
CALORIES 1 SERVING: 50

Circus Carrots

2	cups carrots (finger or julienne cut)	500 mL
2	teaspoons butter	10 mL
2	tablespoons lemon juice	30 mL
2	teaspoons parsley flakes	10 mL

Cook carrots in boiling salted water until tender; keep warm. Melt butter; add lemon juice and parsley flakes. Add warm carrots; toss to coat.

MICROWAVE: Cook carrots in small amount of water on High for 2 minutes. Drain. Add remaining ingredients. Cover. Cook on High for 2 minutes. Toss to mix.

YIELD: 4 servings
EXCHANGE 1 SERVING: ¼ fat, 1 bread
CALORIES 1 SERVING: 59

Candied Carrot Squares

4	carrots	4
1	teaspoon salt	5 mL
2	tablespoons brown sugar replacement	30 mL
2	teaspoons butter	10 mL
½	cup lo-cal cream soda	125 mL

Cut carrots into lengths to make squares. Place carrots in saucepan and cover with water; add salt. Cook until crisp-tender; drain. Place in baking dish. Sprinkle carrots with brown sugar replacement; dot with butter; add cream soda. Bake at 350° F (175° C) for 30 minutes. Turn carrots gently two or three times during baking.

YIELD: 4 servings
EXCHANGE 1 SERVING: 1 bread, ½ fat
CALORIES 1 SERVING: 47

Spinach with Onion

2	pounds fresh spinach	1 kg
2	teaspoons margarine	10 mL
½	cup onion (sliced)	125 mL
	dash nutmeg, thyme, salt, pepper	

Rinse spinach thoroughly; place in top of double boiler and heat until wilted. Drain and chop coarsely. Melt margarine in skillet; add onion. Sauté over high heat until onion is brown on the edges. Add seasonings. Stir to blend. Add spinach and toss to blend.

YIELD: 4 servings
EXCHANGE 1 SERVING: ½ vegetable, ½ fat
CALORIES 1 SERVING: 37

Zucchini Florentine

4	small zucchini	4 small
2	teaspoons margarine	10 mL
1	cup fresh spinach (chopped)	250 mL
1	cup skim milk	250 mL
3	eggs (slightly beaten)	3
1	teaspoon salt	5 mL
¼	teaspoon pepper	1 mL
¼	teaspoon thyme	1 mL
¼	teaspoon paprika	1 mL

Cut zucchini into thin slices. Melt margarine in baking dish; add zucchini. Bake at 400° F (200° C) for 15 minutes. Add spinach. Blend skim milk, eggs, salt, pepper, and thyme. Pour over vegetables. Sprinkle with paprika. Bake at 350° F (175° C) for 40 minutes, or until set.

YIELD: 6 servings
EXCHANGE 1 SERVING: 1 vegetable, ½ medium-fat meat
CALORIES 1 SERVING: 82

Zucchini Wedges

4	small zucchini	4 small
2	teaspoons margarine	10 mL
2	teaspoons onion (grated)	10 mL
1	cube beef bouillon	1 cube
2	tablespoons boiling water	30 mL

Cut zucchini in half lengthwise. Melt margarine in skillet. Add onion and bouillon cube. Press bouillon cube against bottom of skillet to crush. Stir to blend. Place zucchini cut-side down in skillet. Sauté until golden brown; turn. Add boiling water; cover. Cook over low heat for 10 minutes, or until tender.

YIELD: 4 servings
EXCHANGE 1 SERVING: ½ vegetable, ½ fat
CALORIES 1 SERVING: 37

SALADS

Perfect Salad

½	envelope unflavored gelatin	½ envelope
¼	cup cold water	60 mL
1	tablespoon sugar replacement	15 mL
½	teaspoon salt	2 mL
¾	cup hot water	185 mL
1	tablespoon lemon juice	15 mL
2	cucumbers (grated)	2
¼	cup carrot (grated)	60 mL
¼	cup onion (chopped)	60 mL
3	ounces cream cheese	90 g
2	tablespoons lo-cal mayonnaise	30 mL

Dissolve gelatin in cold water. Add gelatin mixture, sugar replacement, and salt to hot water; stir until dissolved. Add lemon juice, cucumbers, carrot, and onion. Beat cream cheese with mayonnaise until smooth. Blend into vegetable mixture. Pour into mold and chill.

YIELD: 8 servings
EXCHANGE 1 SERVING: ½ vegetable, 1 fat
CALORIES 1 SERVING: 73

Mushroom Salad

½	head iceberg lettuce	½ head
½	head Boston lettuce	½ head
1	cucumber	1
½	pound green beans	250 g
½	pound mushrooms	250 g
¼	cup lo-cal French dressing	60 mL

Rinse lettuce. Break into large pieces. Peel and slice cucumber into ¼-inch (6-mm) slices. Rinse green beans; cut beans into 1-inch (2.5-cm) pieces. Place greens, cucumber, and beans into plastic bag or tightly covered container. Store in refrigerator 4 to 6 hours or overnight to crisp. Trim mushroom stems to ¼-inch (6-mm) of cap. (Peel mushrooms if discolored.) Cut mushrooms in thin slices. Just before serving, carefully pat greens, cucumber, and beans dry on towel. Place in wooden bowl; cover with French dressing. Toss to lightly coat all ingredients with dressing. Top with mushrooms.

YIELD: 8 servings
EXCHANGE 1 SERVING: 1 vegetable
CALORIES 1 SERVING: 60

Chinese Salad

1	head Bibb lettuce	1 head
1	head Boston lettuce	1 head
2	stalks Chinese cabbage	2 stalks
8-ounce can water chestnuts		225-g can
8-ounce can bamboo shoots		225-g can
1	cup bean sprouts	250 mL
½	cup Soy French Dressing (page 143)	125 mL

Rinse lettuce and cabbage leaves. Break into bite-size pieces. Place in plastic bag or tightly covered container. Store in refrigerator 4 to 6 hours or overnight to crisp. Drain water chestnuts, bamboo shoots, and bean sprouts. Rinse with cold water. Drain thoroughly. Thinly slice the water chestnuts. Carefully pat greens dry with towel. Place in wooden bowl. Top with water chestnuts, bamboo shoots, and bean sprouts. Cover with Soy French Dressing. Toss lightly until all ingredients are coated.

YIELD: 12 servings
EXCHANGE 1 SERVING: ½ vegetable
CALORIES 1 SERVING: 40

Dandelion Salad

1	cup young dandelion greens	250 mL
1	head iceberg lettuce	1 head
2	tablespoons lo-cal Italian dressing	30 mL
2	tomatoes	2
1	small cucumber	1 small
2	tablespoons lo-cal bleu cheese dressing	30 mL
1	tablespoon skim milk	15 mL

Rinse greens and lettuce. Pat dry with towel. Break into large pieces. Place in large plastic bag. Sprinkle with Italian dressing. Close tightly and store in refrigerator to crisp. Shake occasionally. Peel tomatoes and remove seeds; slice tomato flesh into strips. Peel cucumber; slice into ⅛-inch (3-mm) slices. Place greens, lettuce, tomatoes, and cucumber in wooden bowl. Blend bleu cheese dressing with skim milk. Cover salad with dressing. Toss to coat all ingredients.

YIELD: 6 servings
EXCHANGE 1 SERVING: Negligible
CALORIES 1 SERVING: Negligible

ADDED TOUCH: Top each serving with a few Garlic Bites (page 16). Add exchange and calories for croutons.

Jean's Vegetable Salad

1	cup asparagus, cut into 2-inch (5-cm) pieces	250 mL
1	cup broccoli florets	250 mL
1	cup cauliflowerets	250 mL
½	cup celery (sliced)	125 mL
½	cup cucumber (scored and sliced)	125 mL
1	cup fresh mushrooms (sliced)	250 mL
1	cup green pepper (sliced)	250 mL
½	cup radishes (sliced)	125 mL
10	pitted black olives (sliced)	10
½	cup lo-cal Italian dressing	125 mL

Combine all vegetables in large bowl. Cover with Italian dressing. Marinate overnight. Toss frequently.

YIELD: 7 servings
EXCHANGE 1 SERVING: 1 vegetable
CALORIES 1 SERVING: 45

Radish Salad

1	teaspoon salt	5 mL
1	teaspoon garlic powder	5 mL
1	teaspoon Dijon mustard	5 mL
1	tablespoon wine vinegar	15 mL
2	tablespoons liquid shortening	30 mL
2	teaspoons lemon juice	10 mL
1	watercress (small bunch)	1
½	head iceberg lettuce	½ head
1	bunch red radishes	1 bunch

Combine salt, garlic powder, Dijon mustard, vinegar, liquid shortening, and lemon juice in screw-top jar. Shake to blend. Coarsely chop watercress, lettuce, and radishes; place in salad bowl. Add dressing; toss to blend.

YIELD: 6 servings
EXCHANGE 1 SERVING: 1 fat
CALORIES 1 SERVING: 60

Maude's Green Salad

½	head iceberg lettuce	½ head
½	head Boston lettuce	½ head
½	head chicory	½ head
½	pound spinach	250 g
½	head romaine lettuce	½ head
5	tablespoons lo-cal Italian dressing	75 mL
1	tablespoon Parmesan cheese	15 mL

Rinse and crisp the salad greens. Break iceberg lettuce into bite-size pieces. Carefully pat iceberg dry on towel. Place in large plastic bag. Add 1 tablespoon (15 mL) Italian dressing. Shake lightly until all leaves are covered. Place in strip on medium platter or plate. Repeat with each green. Sprinkle lightly with Parmesan cheese.

YIELD: 10 servings
EXCHANGE: Negligible
CALORIES: Negligible

German Potato Salad

6	slices bacon (crispy fried)	6 slices
1½	cups cold water	375 mL
3	tablespoons flour	45 mL
1	medium onion (chopped)	1 medium
3	tablespoons sugar replacement	45 mL
¼	cup vinegar	60 mL
6	medium boiled potatoes (sliced)	6 medium

Remove excess grease from bacon with paper towel. Break bacon into small pieces. Blend cold water and flour. Pour into saucepan. Add onion, sugar replacement, and vinegar. Heat, stirring, until thickened. Add bacon and potatoes while still warm from boiling and frying.

YIELD: 8 servings
EXCHANGE 1 SERVING: 1 bread, 1 fat
CALORIES 1 SERVING: 113

Swiss Salad

1	small head iceberg lettuce	1 small head
1	head romaine lettuce	1 head
¼	pound fresh spinach	125 g
1	large cucumber	1 large
1	green pepper	1
1	cup cherry tomatoes	250 mL
½	cup lo-cal French dressing	125 mL

Rinse and wash greens. Drain thoroughly. Break into large pieces; place in plastic bag or tightly covered container. Store in refrigerator 4 to 6 hours or overnight to crisp. Score cucumber with tines of fork. Cut into ⅛-inch (3-mm) slices. Cut green pepper into thin rings. Cut cherry tomatoes in half. Just before serving, carefully pat greens dry on towel. Place greens in large wooden bowl; cover with French dressing. Toss greens lightly, coating all leaves with dressing. Top with cucumber, green pepper, and cherry tomatoes. Serve immediately.

YIELD: 16 servings
EXCHANGE 1 SERVING: ½ vegetable
CALORIES 1 SERVING: 32

Marinated Cucumbers

2–3	cucumbers (large)	2–3
1	teaspoon salt	5 mL
1	teaspoon sugar replacement	5 mL
¼	cup vinegar	60 mL
⅛	teaspoon pepper	½ mL

Score cucumbers with tines of fork. Cut into very thin slices. Sprinkle with salt. Chill 2 hours; drain well. Sprinkle with sugar replacement; add vinegar and pepper. Marinate 30 minutes or more before serving.

YIELD: 6 to 8 servings
EXCHANGE: Negligible
CALORIES: Negligible

Asparagus Salad

¼	pound spinach	125 g
1	head romaine lettuce	1 head
10	spears raw asparagus	10 spears
½	head red cabbage	½ head
½	cup celery (sliced)	125 mL
½	cucumber (peeled and sliced)	½
½	cup Lemon French Dressing (page 143)	125 mL

Rinse greens. Break into bite-size pieces. Place in plastic bag or tightly covered container. Store in refrigerator 4 to 6 hours or overnight to crisp. Wash asparagus spears and cut into 2-inch (5-cm) pieces. Shred cabbage as for coleslaw; remove all hard pieces. Just before serving, carefully pat greens dry on towel. Place all ingredients in wooden bowl. Toss lightly to coat all ingredients with Lemon French Dressing.

YIELD: 12 servings
EXCHANGE 1 SERVING: ½ vegetable
CALORIES 1 SERVING: 42

Hot Green Pepper Salad

4	green peppers	4
1	tablespoon butter	15 mL
1	teaspoon oregano	5 mL
½	teaspoon thyme	2 mL
	salt and pepper to taste	
½	cup mushroom pieces	125 mL

Rinse green peppers. Cut them into quarters. Melt butter in skillet. Add seasonings, green peppers, and mushrooms. Cook over low heat for 10 minutes. Serve immediately.

YIELD: 4 servings
EXCHANGE 1 SERVING: 1 vegetable, 1 fat
CALORIES 1 SERVING: 60

Shrimp and Green Bean Salad

2	cups green beans	500 mL
2	cups shrimp	500 mL
½	cup mushrooms (thinly sliced)	125 mL
¼	cup Bay Salad Dressing (page 145)	60 mL
	lettuce leaves	

Rinse and snap green beans. Cook in small amount of boiling salted water until crisp-tender. Drain and cool immediately in ice water; chill. Clean and devein shrimp, or use canned shrimp. Rinse thoroughly under cold water; chill. Combine green beans, shrimp, and mushrooms in bowl. Sprinkle with Bay Salad Dressing. Toss to coat. Chill thoroughly before serving. Serve on lettuce leaves.

YIELD: 4 servings
EXCHANGE 1 SERVING: 1 lean meat, ½ vegetable
CALORIES 1 SERVING: 62

Salmon Salad Plate

1	ounce cold salmon (cooked)	30 g
½	small tomato	½ small
¼	cup carrot sticks	60 mL
¼	green pepper (sliced)	¼
¼	cup eggplant sticks	60 mL
1	egg (hard cooked)	1
1	tablespoon cottage cheese	15 mL
	salt and pepper to taste	
	lettuce leaf	

Chill salmon. Peel tomato and remove seeds; slice tomato flesh into strips. Cook carrot, green pepper, eggplant, and tomato in boiling salted water until crisp-tender. (Remember, the carrot sticks may take more time to cook than the other vegetables.) Drain and chill. Cut egg in half lengthwise. Mash egg yolk with cottage cheese, salt, and pepper; stuff egg white halves. Arrange cooked salmon, vegetables, and stuffed eggs on crisp lettuce leaf.

YIELD: 1 serving
EXCHANGE: 2⅓ lean meat, 1 vegetable
CALORIES: 193

Waldorf Salad

1	cup celery (sliced)	250 mL
1	cup seedless green grapes (halved)	250 mL
1	cup apple (diced)	250 mL
4	dates (pitted and thinly sliced)	4
½	cup walnuts (chopped)	125 mL
¼	cup mayonnaise	60 mL
2	tablespoons dry white wine	30 mL
	lettuce leaves	

Place celery, grapes, apple, dates, and walnuts into bowl. Blend mayonnaise with wine; pour into bowl. Stir to blend with celery, fruit, and walnuts. Use slotted serving spoon to serve, shaking spoon slightly to remove excess dressing. Serve on crisp lettuce leaves.

YIELD: 7 servings
EXCHANGE 1 SERVING: 2 fruit, ¼ vegetable, 1 fat
CALORIES 1 SERVING: 105

Herring Salad Plate

1	ounce salted herring	30 g
½	small onion (thinly sliced)	½ small
¼	cup beets (sliced)	60 mL
	Italian or French dressing	
	lettuce leaf	

Soak herring overnight in water. Remove skin and bones. Cut into
1-inch (2.5-cm) pieces. Place herring, onion, and beets in glass bowl.
Cover with dressing. Marinate 4 to 5 hours or overnight. Drain. (Keep
liquid; it makes a very good salad dressing.) Arrange herring, onion,
and beets on crisp lettuce leaf.

YIELD: 2 servings
EXCHANGE 1 SERVING: ½ lean meat, ¼ vegetable
CALORIES 1 SERVING: 50

Lime Avocado Salad

1	pkg. (⅝ ounce) lo-cal lime gelatin	
	(both envelopes)	1 pkg. (20 g)
1½	cups boiling water	375 mL
3	ounces cream cheese	90 g
½	cup lo-cal whipped topping	
	(prepared)	125 mL
½	cup avocado (cubed)	125 mL
½	cup unsweetened fruit cocktail	125 mL
	vegetable cooking spray	
	shredded lettuce	

Dissolve gelatin in boiling water. Cool to consistency of beaten
egg whites. Beat cream cheese; blend into gelatin mixture. Fold
prepared whipped topping into gelatin mixture. Chill until quite firm.
Fold in avocado and fruit cocktail. Pour into 1-quart (1-L) ring mold
coated with vegetable cooking spray. Chill until set. Serve on bed of
shredded lettuce.

YIELD: 8 servings
EXCHANGE 1 SERVING: ½ vegetable, ½ lean meat, 1 fat
CALORIES 1 SERVING: 78

Cantaloupe Bowl

4	strawberries	4
4	fresh pineapple cubes	4
1	teaspoon sugar replacement	5 mL
¼	6-inch (15-cm) cantaloupe	¼

Sprinkle strawberries and pineapple with sugar replacement. Fill hollow of cantaloupe with fruit mixture.

YIELD: 1 serving
EXCHANGE: 2 fruit
CALORIES: 90

Grapefruit Salad

¼	cup cranberries	60 mL
1½	cups grapefruit sections	375 mL
1	apple (sliced)	1
2	tablespoons raisins	30 mL
½	cup orange juice	125 mL
	lettuce leaves	

Prick cranberries with sharp fork. Combine with remaining ingredients, except lettuce. Marinate 4 to 6 hours or overnight; drain. Serve on crisp lettuce leaves.

YIELD: 5 servings
EXCHANGE 1 SERVING: 1 fruit
CALORIES 1 SERVING: 40

Cranberry Salad

1	pkg. (⅝ ounce) lo-cal lemon gelatin	1 pkg. (20 g)
1	tablespoon sugar replacement	15 mL
1½	cups boiling water	375 mL
1	orange	1
½	cup cranberries	125 mL
½	cup celery (chopped)	125 mL
½	cup apple (chopped)	125 mL

Dissolve gelatin and sugar replacement in boiling water. Cool to consistency of beaten egg whites. Grind orange (with peel) and cranberries; combine with celery and apple. Fold into gelatin mixture. Pour into mold or serving bowl. Chill until firm.

YIELD: 8 servings
EXCHANGE 1 SERVING: ½ fruit
CALORIES 1 SERVING: 24

Queen's Layered Gelatin

1	pkg. (⅝ ounce) lo-cal strawberry gelatin	1 pkg. (20 g)
	Vegetable cooking spray	
1	pkg. (⅝ ounce) lo-cal lemon gelatin	1 pkg. (20 g)
3	ounces cream cheese	90 g
1	cup lo-cal whipped topping (prepared)	250 mL
1	pkg. (⅝ ounce) lo-cal orange gelatin	1 pkg. (20 g)
½	cup unsweetened crushed pineapple (drained)	125 mL
½	cup carrot (grated)	125 mL
	shredded lettuce	

Prepare strawberry gelatin as directed on package. Pour into 2-quart (2-L) mold coated with vegetable cooking spray. Chill until firm. Prepare lemon gelatin as directed on package. Set until consistency of beaten egg whites. Whip cream cheese until light and fluffy. Fold into prepared whipped topping. Fold cream cheese topping into lemon gelatin. Pour over strawberry gelatin in mold. Chill until firm. Prepare orange gelatin as directed on package. Set until consistency of beaten egg whites. Fold in pineapple and carrot. Pour over lemon gelatin in mold. Chill until firm. Serve on bed of shredded lettuce.

YIELD: 8 servings
EXCHANGE 1 SERVING: ½ vegetable, 1 fat
CALORIES 1 SERVING: 57

Blueberry Salad

1½	cups fresh or frozen blueberries	375 mL
2	teaspoons sugar replacement	10 mL
1	envelope unflavored gelatin	1 envelope
2	teaspoons lemon juice	10 mL
1	cup unsweetened crushed pineapple (drained)	250 mL
1	cup lo-cal whipped topping (prepared)	250 mL

Place blueberries in saucepan. Sprinkle with sugar replacement. Allow to rest 30 minutes at room temperature; drain. Add enough boiling water to make 2 cups (500 mL). Sprinkle unflavored gelatin over surface. Stir to dissolve. Cook over low heat for 2 to 3 minutes. Allow to rest until cool. Add lemon juice. Remove ⅓ cup (80 mL) from blueberry mixture. Chill until set; reserve. Fold pineapple into remaining gelatin; chill until firm. Whip reserved gelatin until frothy. Fold in prepared whipped topping. Spread over blueberry gelatin. Chill until set.

YIELD: 4 servings
EXCHANGE 1 SERVING: 1 fruit
CALORIES 1 SERVING: 24

Cabbage–Pineapple Salad

3	cups cabbage (shredded)	750 mL
	1-pound can unsweetened	
	pineapple (diced)	500-g can
2	tablespoons sugar replacement	30 mL
	dash salt	
½	cup lo-cal whipped topping	
	(prepared)	125 mL

Combine cabbage and pineapple with juice from can, sugar replacement, and salt. Stir to dissolve sugar. Allow to rest at room temperature for 1½ to 2 hours. Drain thoroughly. Fold topping into cabbage mixture.

YIELD: 4 servings
EXCHANGE 1 SERVING: ½ fruit
CALORIES 1 SERVING: 28

Note: Lo-cal whipped topping can be made by mixing nondairy whipped topping with water.

Fruit Bowl

¼	cup cantaloupe balls	60 mL
⅛	cup honeydew balls	30 mL
½	cup watermelon balls	125 mL
¼	cup fresh, unsweetened	
	pineapple chunks	60 mL
	salt	
	lo-cal French dressing	
	lettuce	

Sprinkle each fruit with salt and French dressing. Combine all ingredients, except lettuce. Refrigerate 1 to 2 hours. Serve on small bed of lettuce.

YIELD: 1 serving
EXCHANGE: 1 fruit
CALORIES: 40

Fruit Salad

16-ounce can unsweetened apricot halves		500-g can
16-ounce can unsweetened pineapple chunks		500-g can
2	teaspoons lemon juice	10 mL
1	teaspoon cornstarch	5 mL
2	teaspoons sugar replacement	10 mL
1	teaspoon margarine	5 mL
1	apple (chopped)	1
1	banana (sliced)	1
	lo-cal whipped topping	

Drain juice from apricots and pineapple into saucepan; add lemon juice and cornstarch. Cook over low heat to thicken. Remove from heat; add sugar replacement and margarine. Stir to blend; cool slightly. Combine all fruit in bowl. Pour sauce over fruit.

YIELD: 6 servings
EXCHANGE 1 SERVING: 1 fruit
CALORIES 1 SERVING: 53

ADDED TOUCH: Top each serving with a dab of whipped topping.

SAUCES AND SALAD DRESSINGS

Tomato Sauce

firm red tomatoes (or canned tomatoes
without seasonings)

Quarter the tomatoes. Place in large kettle. Push down with hands
or back of spoon to render some juice. Bake at 325° F (165° C) until
soft pulp remains. Spoon into blender. Blend until smooth. Seal in
sterilized jars or freeze.

Creole Sauce

28-ounce can tomatoes		800-g can
1	medium onion (chopped)	1 medium
1	green pepper	1
1	teaspoon paprika	5 mL
¼	teaspoon marjoram	1 mL
	salt and pepper to taste	

Combine all ingredients and cook over low heat for 25 minutes.

YIELD: 2 cups (500 mL)
EXCHANGE: 1 vegetable
CALORIES: 25

Italian Tomato Sauce

6	tomatoes (peeled and cubed)	6
¼	cup green pepper (chopped)	60 mL
¼	cup onion (chopped)	60 mL
2	tablespoons parsley (chopped)	30 mL
1	tablespoon lemon juice	15 mL
	dash oregano, marjoram, thyme, crushed bay leaf, horseradish	
	salt and pepper to taste	

Combine all ingredients in blender. Whip until smooth. Add enough water to make 2 cups (500 mL).

YIELD: 2 cups (500 mL)
EXCHANGE: 2 vegetables
CALORIES: 10

Chili Sauce

	28-ounce can tomatoes	800-g can
1	medium apple	1 medium
1	medium onion	1 medium
1	small green pepper	1 small
1	cup wine vinegar	250 mL
½	cup sugar replacement	125 mL
1	tablespoon salt	15 mL
½	teaspoon ground clove	2 mL
½	teaspoon cinnamon	2 mL
½	teaspoon nutmeg	2 mL

Mash tomatoes; pour into kettle. Grind together apple, onion, green pepper, and vinegar. Add to kettle; cook until thick. Remove from heat. Add sugar replacement and seasonings. Return to heat; cook 5 minutes, stirring constantly.

YIELD: 2 cups (500 mL)
EXCHANGE ½ CUP (125 mL): 1 fruit
CALORIES ½ CUP (125 mL): 45

VARIATIONS FOR ITALIAN DRESSING

To ½ cup (125 mL) lo-cal Italian dressing, add:

ANCHOVY
Mash 1 ounce (30 g) anchovy fillets.

EXCHANGE: 1 meat

BACON
Grind 1 tablespoon (15 mL) Bac-Os®; allow to mellow several hours.

EXCHANGE: ½ fat

PARMESAN
Add 1 tablespoon (15 mL) Parmesan cheese; allow to mellow several hours.

EXCHANGE: ⅛ meat

TOMATO
Add 1 tablespoon (15 mL) tomato purée.

WINE
Add 1 tablespoon (15 mL) dry white or red wine.

CALORIES ½ CUP (125 mL): 24

VARIATIONS FOR FRENCH DRESSING

To ½ cup (125 mL) lo-cal French dressing, add:

AVOCADO
Mash avocado to make 2 tablespoons (30 mL).

EXCHANGE: 1 fat

CHEESE
Mash bleu cheese or Roquefort cheese to make 2 tablespoons (30 mL).

EXCHANGE: ¼ meat

EGG
Crumble 1 hard-cooked egg yolk; combine with dash of hot pepper sauce.

EXCHANGE: 1 meat

LEMON
Add 1 tablespoon (15 mL) lemon juice.

SOY
Add 1 tablespoon (15 mL) soy sauce.

CALORIES ½ CUP (125 mL): 100

VARIATIONS FOR BLEU CHEESE DRESSING

To ½ cup (125 mL) lo-cal bleu cheese dressing, add:

ANCHOVY
Mash 1 ounce (30 g) anchovy fillets.

EXCHANGE: 1 meat

BACON
Grind 1 tablespoon (15 mL) Bac-Os®; allow to mellow several hours.

EXCHANGE: ½ fat

CHIVE
Chop chives to make 2 tablespoons (30 mL); allow to mellow several hours.

HERB
Combine 1 teaspoon (5 mL) each ground parsley, chives, and marjoram.

CALORIES ½ CUP (125 mL): 56

Salad Dressing

1½	cups cold water	375 mL
¼	cup vinegar	60 mL
1½	teaspoons salt	7 mL
1	teaspoon yellow mustard	5 mL
2	tablespoons flour	30 mL
1	egg (well beaten)	1
¼	cup sugar replacement	60 mL
2	teaspoons margarine	10 mL

Combine cold water, vinegar, salt, mustard, flour, and egg in top of double boiler. Stir to blend. Cook until thick. Remove from heat. Add sugar replacement and margarine. Stir to blend.

YIELD: 1 cup (250 mL)
EXCHANGE 2 TABLESPOONS (30 mL): ½ fat
CALORIES 2 TABLESPOONS (30 mL): 31

Sweet Yogurt Dressing

1	cup lo-cal yogurt	250 mL
½	teaspoon mace	2 mL
2	teaspoons sugar replacement	10 mL
	dash salt	
½	cup lo-cal whipped topping (prepared)	125 mL

Drain yogurt; beat until smooth and fluffy. Add mace, sugar replacement, and salt. Beat until blended. Fold in prepared whipped topping. Place in refrigerator until ready to serve. Good on fruit or gelatin salads.

YIELD: 1 cup (250 mL)
EXCHANGE: 1 milk
CALORIES: 100

Herb Yogurt Dressing

1	cup lo-cal yogurt	250 mL
2	tablespoons vinegar	30 mL
1	teaspoon onion (grated)	5 mL
1	teaspoon celery seeds	5 mL
1	teaspoon dry mustard	5 mL
1	teaspoon salt	5 mL
½	teaspoon thyme	2 mL
	salt and pepper to taste	

Beat yogurt until smooth. Add remaining ingredients; blend well. Cover. Allow to rest at least 1 hour before serving.

YIELD: 1 cup (250 mL)
EXCHANGE: I milk
CALORIES: 86

Bay Salad Dressing

3	tablespoons liquid shortening	45 mL
½	cup onion (finely chopped)	125 mL
2	tablespoons fresh parsley (finely chopped)	30 mL
2	tablespoons celery with leaves (finely chopped)	30 mL
1	bay leaf	1
	dash thyme, mace, rosemary	
2	tablespoons white wine	30 mL
1	cup yogurt	250 mL
2	tablespoons skim milk	30 mL
	salt and pepper to taste	

Heat liquid shortening in small skillet. Add onion, parsley, celery, and seasonings. Cook over very low heat, stirring constantly, for

15 minutes. DO NOT ALLOW VEGETABLES TO BURN. Set aside to cool. Add wine; stir to mix. Allow to rest 30 minutes; strain, reserving liquid. Beat yogurt with skim milk. Continue beating, adding wine liquid. Add salt and pepper. Blend.

YIELD: 1 ½ cups (375 mL)
EXCHANGE ¼ CUP (60 mL): ½ vegetable, ½ fat
CALORIES ¼ CUP (60 mL): 44

Tangy Barbecue Sauce

1	cup Chili Sauce (page 141)	250 mL
2	tablespoons lemon juice	30 mL
1	tablespoon Worcestershire sauce	15 mL
1	teaspoon horseradish	5 mL
1	teaspoon Dijon mustard	5 mL
1	tablespoon brown sugar replacement	15 mL
	dash hot pepper sauce, soy sauce, salt, pepper	

Combine all ingredients; stir to blend well.

YIELD: 1 cup (250 mL)
EXCHANGE: 2 fruit
CALORIES: 90

Hollandaise Sauce

1	egg yolk	1
1	tablespoon evaporated (regular or skim) milk	15 mL
⅛	teaspoon salt	½ mL
	dash cayenne pepper	
1	tablespoon lemon juice	15 mL
1	tablespoon margarine	15 mL

In the top of a double boiler, heat egg yolk, evaporated milk, salt, and cayenne pepper until thick. Place over hot water. Beat lemon juice into egg mixture until thick and creamy. Remove double boiler from heat. Add margarine, 1 teaspoon (5 mL) at a time. Beat until margarine is melted and blended in.

YIELD: ½ cup (125 mL)
EXCHANGE: ½ high-fat meat, 3 fat
CALORIES: 213

White Sauce

2	tablespoons margarine	30 mL
1½	tablespoons flour	25 mL
¼	teaspoon salt	1 mL
1	teaspoon Worcestershire sauce	5 mL
1	cup skim milk	250 mL

Melt margarine. Add flour, salt, and Worcestershire sauce. Blend thoroughly. Add skim milk. Cook until slightly thickened.

YIELD: 1 cup (250 mL)
EXCHANGE ½ CUP (125 mL): 1 bread, ½ high-fat meat
CALORIES ½ CUP (125 mL): 190

Orange Sauce

½	teaspoon cornstarch	2 mL
2	tablespoons cold water	30 mL
½	cup orange juice concentrate	125 mL
2	teaspoons unsweetened orange drink mix	10 mL

Dissolve cornstarch in cold water. Add orange juice concentrate and drink mix. Cook over low heat until slightly thickened. Use as glaze on poultry or pork.

YIELD: ½ cup (125 mL)
EXCHANGE: 1 fruit
CALORIES: 52

Teriyaki Marinade

⅓	cup soy sauce	80 mL
2	tablespoons wine vinegar	30 mL
2	tablespoons sugar replacement	30 mL
2	teaspoons salt	10 mL
1	teaspoon ginger (powdered)	5 mL
½	teaspoon garlic powder	2 mL

Blend well. No calories.

SANDWICH SPREADS AND SNACKS

Beef Tongue Spread

6	ounces cooked beef tongue (chopped)	180 g
2	tablespoons Chili Sauce (page 141)	30 mL
1	tablespoon onion (finely chopped)	15 mL

Combine all ingredients; blend well.

YIELD: 1 cup (250 mL)
EXCHANGE ¼ CUP (60 mL): 1 medium-fat meat
CALORIES ¼ CUP (60 mL): 76

Sweet Spread

½	cup margarine	125 mL
1	teaspoon cinnamon	5 mL
1	teaspoon orange rind (grated)	5 mL
½	teaspoon nutmeg	2 mL
2	tablespoons sugar replacement	30 mL

Have margarine at room temperature. Beat until light and fluffy. Add remaining ingredients. Beat until blended.

YIELD: 24 servings
EXCHANGE 1 TEASPOON (5 mL): 1 fat
CALORIES 1 TEASPOON (5 mL): 45

Waldorf Sandwich Spread

¼	cup celery (finely chopped)	60 mL
1	small apple (finely chopped)	1 small
1	tablespoon raisins (finely chopped)	15 mL
6	walnut halves (finely chopped)	6
2	tablespoons Salad Dressing (page 144)	30 mL
	salt to taste	

Combine all ingredients; blend well.

YIELD: ½ cup (125 mL)
EXCHANGE ¼ CUP (60 mL): 1 fruit, 1 fat
CALORIES ¼ CUP (60 mL): 96

Tacos

3	ounces lean ground beef	90 g
	salt and pepper to taste	
1	tablespoon taco sauce	15 mL
3	6-inch (15-cm) taco shells	3
1½	ounces Cheddar cheese (grated)	45 g
1½	tablespoons onion (chopped)	25 mL
1	medium tomato (chopped)	1 medium
1	cup lettuce (shredded)	250 mL

Brown beef over low heat. Add salt and pepper. Drain. Add taco sauce; mix well. Divide beef mixture evenly among warm crisp shells. Top with cheese, onion, tomato, and lettuce.

YIELD: 1 serving
EXCHANGE: 1 bread, 4½ meat, 1 vegetable
CALORIES 1 TACO: 145

Tuna Spread

6½-ounce can tuna (in water)		200-mL can
2	tablespoons onion (finely chopped)	30 mL
2	tablespoons celery (finely chopped)	30 mL
1	tablespoon carrot (finely chopped)	15 mL
¼	cup lo-cal bleu cheese dressing	60 mL
	salt and pepper to taste	

Drain tuna; chop fine. Add remaining ingredients and mix well.

YIELD: 1 cup (250 mL)
EXCHANGE ¼ CUP (60 mL): 1½ lean meat
CALORIES ¼ CUP (60 mL): 48

Blueberry Preserves
(Strawberry, Raspberry)

1	cup fresh or frozen blueberries (unsweetened)	250 mL
1	teaspoon lo-cal pectin	5 mL
1	teaspoon sugar replacement	5 mL

Place blueberries in top of double boiler. Cook over boiling water until soft and juicy. (Crush berries against sides of double boiler.) Add pectin and sugar replacement. Blend in thoroughly. Cook until medium thick. Preserves can also be made with strawberries or raspberries.

MICROWAVE: Place blueberries in glass bowl. Cook on High for 4 minutes until soft and juicy. (Crush berries against sides of bowl.) Add pectin and sugar. Blend in thoroughly. Cook on High 30 seconds.

YIELD: ⅔ cup (160 mL)
EXCHANGE: 1 fruit
CALORIES: 40

Hamburger Relish

2	quarts cucumbers (ground)	2 L
2	onions	2
2	green peppers	2
1	red pepper	1
¼	cup salt	60 mL
2	cups vinegar	500 mL
1	teaspoon mustard seeds	5 mL
1	teaspoon celery seeds	5 mL
1	teaspoon parsley flakes	5 mL
1	teaspoon turmeric	5 mL
2	cups sugar replacement	500 mL

Grind cucumbers, onions, green peppers, and red pepper. Stir in salt. Soak overnight; drain. Combine vinegar, mustard seeds, celery seeds, parsley flakes, and turmeric. Bring to a boil; cook for 10 minutes. Add ground vegetables; cook for 20 minutes. Remove from heat. Add sugar replacement; stir to dissolve. Allow to rest 24 hours; stir often. Drain slightly if too much liquid accumulates. Pack in scalded jars; seal.

YIELD: About 5 pints
EXCHANGE 1 TABLESPOON (15 mL): Negligible
CALORIES 1 TABLESPOON (15 mL): Negligible

Beef Jerky

2	pounds flank steak	1 kg
½	cup soy sauce	125 mL
	lemon pepper to taste	
	garlic salt to taste	

Thoroughly chill flank steak. Cut into ¼ x 8-inch (6 x 20-cm) strips. Combine soy sauce, lemon pepper, and garlic salt. Marinate steak in sauce for 24 hours; drain. Place on broiler pan. Bake at 150° F (65° C) for 10 to 12 hours, or until dry.

EXCHANGE 2 STRIPS: 1 high-fat meat
CALORIES 2 STRIPS: 108

Teeny Pizza

	dough for 1 biscuit	
1	tablespoon Tomato Sauce (page 140)	15 mL
	dash garlic powder, oregano, thyme, salt	
½	ounce meat of your choice	15 g
½	ounce mozzarella cheese (shredded)	15 g

Press or roll biscuit dough flat. Roll edge up or place in individual baking dish. Combine Tomato Sauce and seasonings. Spread over entire surface of biscuit. Top with meat and cheese. Bake at 450° F (230° C) for 10 minutes.

YIELD: 1 serving
EXCHANGE: 1 meat, 1 bread
CALORIES: 150

Wrapped Wiener

1	wiener	1
⅜-in.	strip cheese	1-cm strip
	dough for 1 biscuit	

Make a thin slit in wiener; insert strip of cheese in slit. Roll or pat biscuit dough thin. Place wiener on edge of dough; roll up. Secure by pinching dough together, or use a toothpick. Bake at 375° F (190° C) for 15 minutes, or until golden brown.

YIELD: 1 serving
EXCHANGE: 1¼ meat, 1 bread
CALORIES: 141

Fish Bundles

½	cup Herb-Seasoned Stuffing (page 106)	125 mL
8	ounces Cooked Flaked Fish (page 78)	240 g
1	egg	1

Moisten stuffing with water. Allow to stand 5 minutes, or until soft. (Add extra water if needed.) Blend fish and egg into softened stuffing. Form into 6 patties. Broil for 10 to 15 minutes. Turn once.

YIELD: 6 patties
EXCHANGE 1 PATTY: 1¼ meat, ¼ bread, ⅛ fat
CALORIES 1 PATTY: 45

Garlic Dill Pickles

3	cups water	750 mL
3	cups vinegar	750 mL
½	cup pickling salt	125 mL
	firm medium cucumbers (quartered)	

| 1 | per jar dill head | 1 per jar |
| 1 | per jar garlic clove | 1 per jar |

Combine water, vinegar, and pickling salt. Bring to a boil; cook for 5 minutes. Divide cucumbers, dill, and garlic among three scalded 1 quart (1 L) jars. Fill jars with vinegar mixture. Seal immediately. Ready in 6 to 8 weeks.

EXCHANGE 1 PICKLE: Negligible
CALORIES 1 PICKLE: Negligible

Bread and Butter Pickles

4	quarts cucumbers (sliced)	4 L
5	onions	5
1	quart crushed ice	1 L
⅓	cup salt	80 mL
2	cups vinegar	500 mL
1½	teaspoons turmeric	7 mL
1½	teaspoons celery seeds	7 mL
2	teaspoons mustard seeds	10 mL
1	teaspoon ginger	5 mL
1½	cups sugar replacement	375 mL

Slice cucumbers and onions; place in large saucepan. Mix ice and salt; stir into cucumbers and onions. Cover. Chill for 5 to 6 hours. Drain; remove ice. Combine vinegar and seasonings. Bring to a boil; simmer for 5 minutes. Add sugar replacement; stir to dissolve. Add drained cucumbers and onions. Bring to a boil. Put into scalded jars and seal.

YIELD: 4 to 5 pints
EXCHANGE 1 TABLESPOON (15 mL): Negligible
CALORIES 1 TABLESPOON (15 mL): Negligible

Dill Midgets

1	head dill	1 head
20–25	firm midget cucumbers	20–25
½	teaspoon alum	2 mL
2	teaspoons pickling salt	10 mL
½	cup white vinegar	125 mL

Scald 1 pint (½ L) jar. Push dill head to bottom of jar. Fill with midgets. Add alum and pickling salt. Pour vinegar over top. Add enough cold water to fill jar; seal. Shake vigorously. Ready in 8 to 10 weeks.

YIELD: 20 to 25 pickles
EXCHANGE 1 PICKLE: Negligible
CALORIES 1 PICKLE: Negligible

Russian Teasicles

2	quarts water	2 L
1	cinnamon stick	1
3	whole cloves	3
2	tablespoons black tea leaves	30 mL
	6-ounce can frozen lemon juice (unsweetened)	180-mL can
	6-ounce can frozen orange juice	180-mL can
½	cup sugar replacement	125 mL

Combine water, cinnamon stick, whole cloves, and black tea leaves in large kettle. Bring to a boil; reduce heat and simmer for 15 to 20 minutes. Strain; cool slightly. Add frozen concentrates and sugar replacement. Stir to dissolve. Pour into freezer stick trays; freeze.

YIELD: about 38 popsicles
EXCHANGE 1 POPSICLE: ½ fruit
CALORIES 1 POPSICLE: 5

Egg Nog

1	egg (well beaten)	1
2	teaspoons sugar replacement	10 mL
	dash salt, vanilla extract	
¾	cup cold milk	185 mL
	dash nutmeg to taste	

Combine egg with sugar replacement and salt. Add vanilla extract and cold milk. Beat well. Pour into glass or mug; sprinkle with nutmeg.

YIELD: 1 serving
EXCHANGE: 1 meat, 1 milk
CALORIES: 148

SPECIAL DESSERT SECTION

CAKES, TORTS, AND CAKE ROLLS

Strawberry Topping
(Blueberry, Raspberry)

2	cups fresh or frozen strawberries (unsweetened)	500 mL
1½	teaspoons cornstarch	7 mL
¼	cup cold water	60 mL
2	teaspoons sugar replacement	10 mL

Place strawberries in top of double boiler. Cook over boiling water until soft and juicy. Blend cornstarch and cold water. Add to strawberries. Cook until clear and slightly thickened. Remove from heat; add sugar replacement. Cool. Topping can also be made with blueberries or raspberries.

YIELD: 1½ cups (375 mL)
EXCHANGE ½ CUP (125 mL): 1 fruit
CALORIES ½ CUP (125 mL): 40

Strawberry Shortcake

	dough for 1 biscuit	
½	cup Strawberry Topping	125 mL
¼	cup fresh strawberries (halved)	60 mL
2	tablespoons lo-cal whipped topping (prepared)	30 mL

Bake biscuit as directed on package. Cool. Cut in half. Layer biscuit, half of the Strawberry Topping, and half of the strawberries; repeat. Top with prepared whipped topping.

YIELD: 1 serving
EXCHANGE: 1 bread, 1 ½ fruit
CALORIES: 100

Banana Cake Roll

4	eggs (separated)	4
10	tablespoons granulated sugar replacement	150 mL
½	teaspoon vanilla extract	2 mL
⅔	cup cake flour (sifted)	160 mL
1	teaspoon baking powder	5 mL
¼	teaspoon salt	1 mL
	vegetable cooking spray	
1	package loc-cal banana pudding (prepared)	1 package
	Chocolate Drizzle (opposite)	

Beat egg yolks until thick and lemon colored; gradually beat in 3 tablespoons (45 mL) of the sugar replacement. Add vanilla extract. Beat egg whites to soft peaks; gradually beat in the remaining sugar replacement; beat until stiff peaks form. Fold yolks into whites. Sift together cake flour, baking powder, and salt. Fold into egg mixture. Spread batter into 15½ x 10½ x 1-inch (39 x 25 x 3-cm) jelly-roll pan (coated with vegetable cooking spray and lightly floured). Bake at 375° F (190° C) for 10 to 15 minutes, or until done. Loosen sides and turn out on towel lightly sprinkled with a mixture of flour and sugar replacement. Roll up cake and towel from narrow end. Cool completely; unroll. Spread evenly with prepared banana pudding. Roll up. Frost with Chocolate Drizzle.

YIELD: 10 servings
EXCHANGE 1 SERVING: 1 bread, ¼ milk
CALORIES 1 SERVING: 62

Chocolate Drizzle

2	teaspoons cornstarch	10 mL
¼	cup cold water	60 mL
	dash salt	
1	ounce unsweetened chocolate	30 g
⅓	cup sugar replacement	80 mL
½	teaspoon butter	2 mL

Blend cornstarch and cold water. Pour into small saucepan. Add salt and chocolate. Cook on low heat until chocolate melts and mixture is thick. Remove from heat. Stir in sugar replacement. Blend in butter.

YIELD: ⅓ cup (80 mL)
EXCHANGE: Negligible
CALORIES: Negligible

Rich Chocolate Cake

1⅓	cups cake flour	330 mL
⅓	cup unsweetened cocoa powder	80 mL
¼	teaspoon baking powder	1 mL
¼	teaspoon baking soda	1 mL
	pinch salt (optional)	
½	cup egg substitute	125 mL
1	teaspoon vanilla extract	5 mL
1	tablespoon raspberry liqueur	15 mL
½	cup nonfat buttermilk	125 mL
4	tablespoons margarine or butter	60 mL
2	tablespoons prune purée	30 mL
15	packets concentrated acesulfame-K	15 packets
3	tablespoons sugar	45 mL
6	egg whites	6
¼	teaspoon cream of tartar	1 mL
½	cup frozen raspberries	125 mL
½	teaspoon concentrated aspartame	2 mL

Sift the first five ingredients together twice; set aside. Combine the egg substitute and vanilla extract, raspberry liqueur, and buttermilk. Using an electric mixer, cream the margarine or butter and the prune purée. Add acesulfame-K and sugar and beat well. Gradually add the egg substitute alternately with the flour mixture. Beat until well combined. Beat the egg whites until stiff. Add the cream of tartar and continue beating. Add a small amount of egg whites to the batter to lighten it. With a rubber spatula, fold in the remaining beaten whites. Pour into two 8-inch (20-cm) round cake pans that have been coated with nonstick cooking spray.

Bake in a preheated 350° F (175° C) oven for 30 to 35 minutes. Cool, then invert onto a plate. Combine the raspberries and aspartame in a food processor to make raspberry purée. Spread raspberry purée over the top of one layer. Put the other layer on top and cover with raspberry purée. Decorate top with whole raspberries if desired.

YIELD: 10 servings
EXCHANGES: 2 bread, ½ fat
CALORIES: 189

Angel Food Cake

1	cup flour	250 mL
¼	cup sugar	60 mL
3	packets concentrated acesulfame-K	3 packets
1½	cups egg whites (12)	375 mL
1½	teaspoons cream of tartar	7 mL
¼	teaspoon salt	1 mL
¼	cup sugar	60 mL
4	packets concentrated acesulfame-K	4 packets
1½	teaspoons vanilla extract	7 mL
½	teaspoon almond extract	2 mL

Sift together the flour, ¼ cup (60 mL) of sugar, and 3 packets of acesulfame-K. Set aside. In a large mixing bowl, combine the egg whites, cream of tartar, and salt. With an electric mixer, beat until foamy. Mix together ¼ cup (60 mL) of sugar and 4 more packets of the acesulfame-K. Gradually add this mixture, a tablespoon (15 mL) at a time, to the egg whites. Continue beating until stiff peaks form. Fold in the vanilla and almond extracts. Sprinkle the flour mixture over the beaten egg whites. Fold gently just until the flour disappears. Fold the batter into an ungreased 10 x 4-inch (25 x 10-cm) tube pan.

Bake in a 375° F (190° C) oven for 30 to 35 minutes, until no imprint remains when finger lightly touches the top of the cake. The top should be golden brown. To cool, turn the baked cake over. For best results, stand the tube pan on a custard cup or put a bottle in the center hole to hold the top away from the counter so circulation will occur. Remove the cake from the pan only after it is thoroughly cooled. Drizzle with bittersweet topping, fruit topping, or sliced fresh fruit.

YIELD: 24 slices
EXCHANGE: ½ bread
CALORIES: 42
(PLUS CALORIES AND EXCHANGES FOR TOPPING)

Chocolate Éclair Cake

Dough

1	cup water	250 mL
½	cup canola oil	125 mL
1	cup flour	250 mL
4	eggs	4
1	teaspoon butter-flavored extract	5 mL

Filling

2	8-ounce pkgs. sugar-free vanilla pudding	2 244-g pkgs.
2½	cups skim milk	625 mL
¾	cup prepared sugar-free, low-fat whipped topping from mix	185 mL

Topping

6	tablespoons unsweetened cocoa powder	90 mL
2	tablespoons canola oil	30 mL
2	tablespoons skim milk	30 mL
¾	cup aspartame	185 mL
1	teaspoon vanilla extract	5 mL
	extra milk, if needed	
1	teaspoon butter-flavored extract	5 mL

TO MAKE THE DOUGH: Heat the water and oil to a rolling boil. Stir in the flour over low heat until the mixture forms a ball. Remove from the heat. Using an electric mixer, beat in the eggs thoroughly, one at a time. Put in the butter extract. Spoon onto an ungreased cookie sheet in the shape of a ring or wreath. Bake until golden brown and dry at 400° F (200° C) for 35 to 40 minutes. Cool away from drafts. Slice in half horizontally. Just before serving, add the filling by removing the top half, adding the filling, and replacing the top. Add the topping.

TO MAKE THE FILLING: Whisk the pudding and milk until the mixture thickens. Fold in the whipped topping.

TO MAKE THE TOPPING: Melt the cocoa powder with the oil and milk. Cool. Add the aspartame and vanilla and beat until the mixture is the desired consistency. Add a little extra milk if necessary, one teaspoon at a time. Drizzle on top of the cake.

YIELD: 24 servings
EXCHANGE: 1 bread, 1 fat
CALORIES: 100

Banana Tea Bread

½	cup egg substitute	125 mL
1	cup ripe banana, mashed	250 mL
1	teaspoon vanilla extract	5 mL
2	cups flour	500 mL
½	teaspoon salt	2 mL
1	teaspoon baking soda	5 mL
2	tablespoons sugar	30 mL
6	packets concentrated acesulfame-K	6 packets

Glaze

2	tablespoons boiling water	30 mL
4	teaspoons concentrated aspartame	20 mL

Beat the egg substitute with a wire whisk; add the mashed banana and vanilla extract. Sift together the flour, salt, baking soda, sugar, and acesulfame-K. Add these dry ingredients to the egg–banana mixture and stir. Turn the mixture into a loaf pan that has been coated with nonstick cooking spray. Bake in a preheated 350° F (175° C) oven for 40 minutes.

After the bread is out of the oven, poke holes all over the top using a fork. Combine boiling water and the aspartame; use a pastry brush to cover the top with glaze, letting the glaze sink into the holes.

YIELD: 20 servings
EXCHANGE: 1 bread
CALORIES: 66

Mocha Chocolate Roll

1	cup sifted cake flour	250 mL
¼	cup unsweetened cocoa powder	60 mL
1	teaspoon baking powder	5 mL
3	eggs	3
¼	cup sugar	60 mL
3	packets concentrated acesulfame-K	3 packets
⅓	cup cold coffee	80 mL
1	teaspoon vanilla extract	5 mL

Filling

1	package sugar-free whipped topping mix	1 package
½	cup cold, very strong coffee	125 mL

Spray a 15 x 10 x 1-inch (37 x 25 x 3-cm) jelly-roll pan; line the bottom with wax paper; spray the paper. Sift the flour, cocoa, and baking powder together. With an electric mixer, beat the eggs in a medium bowl until thick and creamy and light in color. Gradually add the sugar and acesulfame-K, beating constantly until the mixture is very thick. Stir in the coffee and vanilla extract. Fold in the flour mixture. Spread the batter evenly in a prepared pan.

Bake in a 350° F (175° C) oven for 12 minutes or until the center springs back when pressed lightly with a fingertip. Loosen the cake around the edges with a knife; invert the pan onto a clean tea towel. Peel off the wax paper. Starting at the short end, roll up the cake and towel together. Place the roll, seam-side down, on a wire rack; cool completely.

To make the filling, follow the directions for the whipped topping mix on the package, but use the cold coffee instead of water. When the cake is cool, unroll it carefully. Spread it evenly with filling. To start rerolling, lift the cake with the end of the towel. Place it, seam-side down, on a serving plate.

YIELD: 20 servings
EXCHANGE: ½ bread, ½ fat
CALORIES: 70

French Pastry Cake

½	cup margarine or butter	125 mL
½	cup nonfat cream cheese	125 mL
¼	cup sugar	60 mL
½	cup measures-like-sugar saccharin	125 mL
2	eggs or equivalent egg substitute	2
1	cup nonfat sour cream	250 mL
1	cup nonfat mayonnaise	250 mL
1	tablespoon vanilla extract	15 mL
2	cups flour	500 mL
1	teaspoon baking powder	5 mL
1	teaspoon baking soda	5 mL

Cinnamon Mixture

1	tablespoon cinnamon	15 mL
2	packets concentrated acesulfame-K	2 packets
½	cup chopped almonds	125 mL

Cream margarine or butter and cream cheese with sugar and saccharin. Add the eggs, sour cream, mayonnaise, and vanilla extract; beat well. Mix the flour, baking powder, and baking soda and add to the batter. Put half the batter into a tube pan or bundt pan coated with nonstick cooking spray. Mix together the cinnamon, acesulfame-K, and chopped almonds. Sprinkle half the cinnamon mixture on top of the batter in the pan, then add the rest of the batter. Sprinkle the rest of the cinnamon mixture on top of the batter. Bake at 350° F (175° C) 60 to 75 minutes or until the top is light brown and the cake pulls away from the pan.

YIELD: 20 servings
EXCHANGE: 1 fat, 1 bread
CALORIES: 155

CHEESECAKES

Granola Cheesecake

Crust

¼	cup margarine or butter, melted	60 mL
1	tablespoon water	15 mL
3	packets concentrated acesulfame-K	3 packets
1	cup granola topping	250 mL

Filling

8	ounces nonfat cream cheese, softened	250 mL
1	cup nonfat cottage cheese, drained	250 mL
½	cup egg substitute or 2 eggs	125 mL
3	packets concentrated acesulfame-K	3 packets
1	teaspoon vanilla extract	5 mL
1	tablespoon flour	15 mL

Topping

⅓	cup granola topping	80 mL

Stir the crust ingredients together and press the mixture into the bottom of a 9-inch (23-cm) springform pan. Set aside. Beat the filling ingredients together until smooth. Spoon this carefully over the crust. Sprinkle the top with granola topping. Bake in a 375° F (190° C) oven for 40 minutes or until set. Cool before removing cake from the pan.

YIELD: 10 servings
EXCHANGE: 1 meat
CALORIES: 88

Healthy Cheesecake

¼	cup graham cracker crumbs	60 mL
2	cups yogurt cheese*	500 mL
2	teaspoons vanilla extract	10 mL
½	cup egg substitute	125 mL
2	tablespoons cornstarch	30 mL
6	packets concentrated acesulfame-K	6 packets

Topping

½	cup nonfat sour cream	125 mL
2	teaspoons sugar	10 mL
2	teaspoons concentrated acesulfame-K	10 mL
1	teaspoon vanilla extract	5 mL

Spray a 9-inch (23-cm) springform pan with nonstick cooking spray. Sprinkle it evenly with graham cracker crumbs. Set aside.

Use an electric mixer to combine the next five ingredients. Beat until creamy. Pour the mixture onto the crumbs. Bake in a preheated 325° F (165° C) oven for 35 minutes. Remove from the oven and let cool. Refrigerate. Combine the topping ingredients and pour the mixture over the baked, chilled cheesecake. Return it to the oven for 10 minutes. Chill. Run a knife around the edge of the pan to loosen the cheesecake.

YIELD: 12 servings
EXCHANGE: ½ bread, ⅓ medium-fat meat
CALORIES: 49

Yogurt cheese is made by letting yogurt drip through cheesecloth overnight in the refrigerator.

Apple Cheesecake

1	pound nonfat cottage cheese	500 g
⅔	cup nonfat sour cream	160 mL
4	teaspoons fructose	20 mL
2	eggs	2
1	tablespoon all-purpose flour	15 mL
½	teaspoon nutmeg	2 mL
pinch cinnamon		pinch
1	juice of one lemon	1
4	small apples, peeled, cored, and sliced into half moons	4
	Graham Cracker Crust (page 173) (optional)	

Spray a 9-inch (23-cm) springform pan with nonstick cooking spray. Sprinkle it evenly with graham cracker crumbs. Set aside.

Beat the cottage cheese, sour cream, fructose, eggs, flour, nutmeg, and cinnamon until smooth. Stir in the lemon juice. Spread half the apples on the bottom, over a crust if you like. Pour the cottage cheese mixture over the apples. Top with the remaining apples. Bake in a preheated oven at 375° F (190° C) or until set. Cool completely.

YIELD: 10 servings
EXCHANGE: ⅓ fruit, ½ lean meat, ¼ bread
CALORIES: 101
(PLUS CALORIES AND EXCHANGES FOR CRUST)

Cheesecake with Jelly Glaze

1	8-ounce pkg. nonfat cream cheese	1 250-mL pkg.
1	cup nonfat yogurt sweetened with aspartame	250 mL
1	package unsweetened gelatin	1 package
¼	cup water	60 mL

1	tablespoon measures-like-sugar aspartame	15 mL
1	cup fresh fruit, or canned, no sugar added	250 mL
3	tablespoons jelly, made with Splenda®	45 mL

Combine the cream cheese and yogurt and beat until smooth. In a small saucepan, sprinkle the gelatin into the water; let soften for 2 minutes. Over low heat, stir to dissolve the gelatin. Remove from the heat and add to cream cheese mixture. Add the aspartame. With an electric mixer, beat until smooth. Pour into a crust of your choice (a Graham Cracker Crust, page 173, is traditional). Arrange the fruit on top. MICROWAVE the jelly for 30 seconds or heat in a saucepan over low heat. When jelly is liquefied, use a pastry brush to glaze the top of the cheesecake.

YIELD: 8 servings
EXCHANGE: 1 milk
CALORIES: 60
(PLUS CALORIES AND EXCHANGES FOR CRUST)

Pumpkin Cheesecake

1	pound nonfat cream cheese	500 g
12	teaspoons fructose	60 mL
¼	cup egg substitute	60 mL
1	16-ounce can pumpkin	1 488-mL can
1½	teaspoons cinnamon	7 mL
1	teaspoon allspice	5 mL
¼	teaspoon ginger	1 mL
¼	teaspoon mace	1 mL
1	unbaked crust, preferably Graham Cracker Crust (page 173) 1	

Spray an 8-inch (20-cm) springform pan with nonstick vegetable cooking spray. Line the bottom of the sprayed pan with crust, if desired. Beat the cream cheese, fructose, and egg substitute until smooth. Beat the pumpkin and spices into the cheese mixture. Spoon the filling into the crust, if used. Bake in a preheated 350° F (175° C) oven for 45 minutes or until set. Cool the cake completely before removing it from the pan.

YIELD: 10 servings
EXCHANGE: 1 milk
CALORIES: 82
(PLUS CALORIES AND EXCHANGES FOR CRUST)

Ricotta Pie

2	pounds fat-free ricotta	1 kg
6	eggs	6
⅓	cup sugar	80 mL
⅓	cup measures-like-sugar saccharin	80 mL
2	teaspoons vanilla extract	10 mL
2	teaspoons butter-flavored extract	10 mL
1	teaspoon cinnamon	5 mL

With an electric mixer, beat all the ingredients except the cinnamon until smooth. Pour the batter into a 10-inch (25-cm) pie crust of your choice. Sprinkle with cinnamon. Bake at 350° F (175° C) for 50 to 60 minutes until a knife inserted comes out clean. Cool. Refrigerate.

YIELD: 8 servings
EXCHANGE: 1½ milk, 1 meat
CALORIES: 159
(PLUS CALORIES AND EXCHANGES FOR CRUST)

No-Bake Orange Cheesecake

Graham Cracker Crust

1	cup finely crushed graham cracker crumbs	250 mL
3	tablespoons melted margarine or butter	45 mL

TO MAKE THE CRUST: Mix the graham cracker crumbs and margarine. Spread this over the bottom and a little up the sides of a 9-inch (23-cm) springform pan. Freeze the crust while mixing the filling.

Cheesecake Filling

¼	cup cold water	60 mL
1	envelope unflavored gelatin	1 envelope
16	ounces nonfat cream cheese, at room temperature	500 g
¼	cup sugar	60 mL
6	packets concentrated acesulfame-K	6 packets
1	cup nonfat sour cream	250 mL
¾	cup freshly squeezed orange juice	185 mL
1	teaspoon freshly grated orange peel	5 mL
2	teaspoons orange flavoring	10 mL

Topping

3	navel oranges, peeled, bitter parts removed	3

TO MAKE THE FILLING: Put the water in a small saucepan and sprinkle the gelatin on top. After 1 minute, turn the heat on low and, stirring constantly, heat for 2–3 minutes until the gelatin is dissolved. Remove from heat.

With an electric mixer, beat the cream cheese, sugar, and acesulfame-K in a large bowl. When the mixture is fluffy, add the sour cream and beat well. Mix in the orange juice, gelatin, peel, and flavoring. Pour into a chilled crust. Refrigerate for 4 to 6 hours until firm.

Before serving, run a thin knife around the edge of the cake to loosen it. Remove the springform from the outside. Top the cake with sliced oranges.

YIELD: 12 servings
EXCHANGE: 1 bread, ½ fat, ½ milk
CALORIES: 164

Creamy Amaretto Cheesecake

2	8-ounce pkgs. nonfat cream cheese	2 244-g pkgs.
2	tablespoons cornstarch	30 mL
2	teaspoons concentrated acesulfame-K	10 mL
2	tablespoons sugar	30 mL
¼	cup Amaretto	60 mL
1	teaspoon vanilla extract	5 mL
½	cup egg substitute	125 mL
1	Graham Cracker Crust (page 173, optional)	1
	fresh fruit (optional)	

Cream the first six ingredients together. Pour in the egg substitute and beat with an electric mixer until creamy. Pour the batter into an 8-inch (20-cm) Graham Cracker Crust, or lightly coat an 8-inch (20-cm) pie plate with nonfat vegetable spray. Bake in a preheated 325° F (165° C) oven for 35 minutes. Chill. Before serving, top with fruit, if desired.

YIELD: 8 servings
EXCHANGE: 1 milk
CALORIES: 108
(PLUS CALORIES AND EXCHANGES FOR GRAHAM CRACKER CRUST)

Strawberry Cream Cheese Tarts

6	ounces nonfat cream cheese	180 g
¾	cup nonfat cottage cheese	185 mL
⅔	cup nonfat sour cream	160 mL
3	eggs separated	3
7	teaspoons fructose	35 mL
1	Graham Cracker Crust (page 173), pressed into 18 mini tart pans	1

To prepare the filling, beat the cream cheese, cottage cheese, sour cream, egg yolks, and fructose in a large bowl until smooth. In another bowl, beat the egg whites until soft peaks form; fold them into the cheese mixture. Spoon the filling into the prepared crusts. Chill until set. Garnish with Strawberry Topping (page 159).

YIELD: 18 tarts
EXCHANGE: ½ milk, 1 bread (for crust)
CALORIES: 44

Marble Cheesecake

2	cups nonfat ricotta cheese	500 mL
8	ounces nonfat cream cheese	250 g
¼	cup egg substitute	60 mL
3	egg whites	3
2	tablespoons sugar	30 mL
12	packets concentrated acesulfame-K	12 packets
1	tablespoon vanilla extract	15 mL
1½	teaspoons lemon juice	7 mL
3	tablespoons cocoa	45 mL
3	tablespoons water	45 mL
2	packets concentrated acesulfame-K	2 packets
3	tablespoons crumbs made from chocolate cookies sweetened with fructose	45 mL

Put the ricotta cheese in a food processor or blender and process for a full minute. Soften the cream cheese in a MICROWAVE oven for 30 seconds. Add it to the food processor with the egg substitute, egg whites, sugar, 12 packets of acesulfame-K, vanilla extract, and lemon juice. Process to combine. In a medium bowl, whisk together the cocoa, water, and 2 packets of acesulfame-K.

Pour approximately 1 cup (250 mL) cheese batter from the food processor into the cocoa. Whisk to combine. Set aside this "chocolate" batter. Then take a 9-inch (23-cm) springform baking pan that has been sprayed with nonstick vegetable cooking spray. Pour most of the white batter into this prepared pan. Pour all the chocolate batter in the center on top of the white batter. There will be a white ring all around the edge of the pan. Carefully pour the rest of the white batter into the center of the chocolate batter. Use a knife to marble the batters by making an "S" curve through the batter. Do not mix completely.

Place the springform pan in the center of a baking pan. Slowly and carefully pour boiling water into the outer baking pan, smoothing the batter in the springform pan. (This hot-water bath will help the cheesecake bake like a custard.) Bake in a preheated 325° F (165° C) oven for 50 minutes or until it starts to shrink away from the sides of the pan. Remove the cake from the hot-water bath and chill it completely overnight. Press chocolate cookie crumbs onto the sides of the cake.

YIELD: 16 servings
EXCHANGE: ½ milk
CALORIES: 57

COOKIES, SQUARES, AND OTHER FINGER FOOD

Oatmeal Cookies

1	cup flour	250 mL
½	teaspoon salt	2 mL
½	teaspoon baking powder	2 mL
¼	teaspoon baking soda	1 mL
½	teaspoon cinnamon	2 mL
½	teaspoon nutmeg	2 mL
½	cup raisins	125 mL
1½	cups oatmeal	375 mL
½	cup sugar replacement	125 mL
½	cup margarine (melted)	125 mL
1	egg	1
½	cup skim milk	125 mL

Combine flour, salt, baking powder, baking soda, cinnamon, nutmeg, raisins, and oatmeal. Mix thoroughly. Beat in sugar replacement, melted margarine, egg, and skim milk. (Add small amount of water if dough is too stiff.) Drop by teaspoonfuls onto cookie sheet. Bake at 400° F (200° C) for 10 minutes.

YIELD: 36 cookies
EXCHANGE 1 COOKIE: ½ bread, ¼ fat
CALORIES 1 COOKIE: 37

Cookie Cutter Cookies

1	cup margarine or butter	250 mL
¼	cup sugar	60 mL
6	packets concentrated acesulfame-K	6 packets
2½	cups flour	625 mL
1	teaspoon baking soda	5 mL
1	teaspoon cream of tartar	5 mL
1	teaspoon vanilla extract	5 mL
1	teaspoon almond extract	5 mL
1	egg or equivalent egg substitute	1

Cream the margarine and sugar. Stir in the rest of the ingredients one at a time in the order listed. Form the dough into a ball, wrap it in plastic wrap, and refrigerate it for at least two hours. Cut the dough into thirds. Roll each third ⅛-inch (3-mm) thick on a lightly floured board. Cut the dough into shapes with cookie cutters. Place the cookies onto ungreased cookie sheets. Bake at 400° F (200° C) for 5 to 8 minutes.

YIELD: 100 small cookies
EXCHANGE: ½ fat
CALORIES: 29

Pecan Tea Cookies

2	cups finely chopped pecans	500 mL
1	cup margarine	250 mL
2	tablespoons sugar	30 mL
2	packets concentrated acesulfame-K	2 packets
2	cups flour	500 mL
1	teaspoon vanilla extract	5 mL
1	tablespoon water	15 mL

Mix all the ingredients together. Chill for half an hour. Shape into small balls. Place on a cookie sheet coated with nonstick cooking spray. Bake in a 350° F (175° C) oven for 12 to 13 minutes until light brown.

YIELD: 80 cookies
EXCHANGE: 1 fat
CALORIES: 50

Cinnamon Crescents

1	cup margarine or butter	250 mL
2	cups flour, sifted	500 mL
1	egg yolk	1
¾	cup nonfat sour cream	185 mL
3	tablespoons sugar	45 mL
3	packets concentrated acesulfame-K	3 packets
¾	cup finely chopped walnuts	185 mL
2	teaspoons cinnamon	10 mL
1	egg white, slightly beaten in 1 tablespoon (15 mL) water	1

Cut the margarine into the flour until the mixture resembles coarse crumbs. Stir in the egg yolk and sour cream. Form a ball. Cover with plastic wrap and chill for two hours. Combine the sugar, acesulfame-K, walnuts, and cinnamon. Divide the dough into fourths. Roll each into an 11-inch (28-cm) circle. Sprinkle each circle with a quarter of the sugar mixture. Cut into 16 wedges. Roll up the wedges, starting at the widest end. Place the rolls on an ungreased cookie sheet. Brush with egg white and water. Bake in a 350° F (175° C) oven for 20 minutes or until golden brown. Cool on wire racks.

YIELD: 48 cookies
EXCHANGE: ½ bread, ½ fat
CALORIES: 70

Snickerdoodles

1	cup margarine or butter	250 mL
¼	cup sugar	60 mL
6	packets concentrated acesulfame-K	6 packets
2	eggs	2
1	teaspoon vanilla extract	5 mL
2⅔	cups flour, sifted	660 mL
2	teaspoons cream of tartar	10 mL
1	teaspoon baking soda	5 mL

Coating

2	tablespoons sugar	30 mL
1	teaspoon cinnamon	5 mL

Beat the margarine until light. Add the sugar and acesulfame-K and beat until fluffy. Beat in the eggs and vanilla. Sift together the flour, cream of tartar, and baking soda. Add this to the margarine mixture.

Combine the sugar and cinnamon in a separate bowl. With floured hands, shape the dough into small balls about 1 inch (2.5 cm) and roll each one in the sugar–cinnamon mixture. Place each 2 inches (5 cm) apart on an ungreased baking sheet. Bake at 400° F (200° C) for 8–10 minutes. Cool on wire racks.

YIELD: 6 dozen cookies
EXCHANGE: ½ fat
CALORIES: 44

Peanut Butter Cookies

2	tablespoons margarine or butter	30 mL
½	cup peanut butter	125 mL
¼	cup sugar	60 mL
3	packets concentrated acesulfame-K	3 packets
1	egg or egg substitute, beaten	1
2	cups flour	500 mL
4	teaspoons baking powder	20 mL
⅓	cup milk	80 mL

Cream the margarine thoroughly, add the peanut butter, and cream together, then blend in the sugar and acesulfame-K. Add the beaten egg. Mix and sift the dry ingredients and add them alternately to the creamed mixture with the milk. Roll into small balls and place on a baking sheet coated with nonstick cooking spray. Flatten with the bottom of a glass dipped in flour. Then, using a fork, make criss-cross impressions in each cookie. Bake in a 400° F (200° C) oven for 7 minutes.

YIELD: 70 cookies
EXCHANGE: Free
CALORIES: 27

Brownies

½	cup flour	125 mL
½	teaspoon baking powder	2 mL
½	teaspoon salt	2 mL
3	ounces unsweetened chocolate (melted)	90 g
½	cup shortening (soft)	125 mL
2	eggs (beaten)	2
2	tablespoons granulated sugar	30 mL
1½	cups sugar replacement	375 mL
1	teaspoon vanilla extract	5 mL

Combine all ingredients. Beat vigorously until well blended. Spread mixture into greased 8-inch (20-cm) square pan. Bake at 350° F (175° C) for 30 to 35 minutes. Cut into 2-inch (5-cm) squares.

MICROWAVE: Cook on Medium for 8 to 10 minutes, or until puffed and dry on top. Cut into 2-inch (5-cm) squares.

YIELD: 16 brownies
EXCHANGE 1 BROWNIE: 1½ bread, 1½ fat
CALORIES 1 BROWNIE: 136

Cranberry Bars

1¼	cups flour	310 mL
1	cup cereal crumbs	250 mL
¼	teaspoon salt	1 mL
¼	cup cold butter	60 mL
1	egg (beaten)	1
4	tablespoons sugar replacement	60 mL
2	tablespoons nuts	30 mL
	vegetable cooking spray	
1	orange	1
1½	cups cranberries	375 mL
⅓	cup water	80 mL
2	tablespoons cornstarch	30 mL
½	teaspoon ground allspice	2 mL

Combine flour, cereal crumbs, and salt in mixing bowl. Cut in cold butter until mixture resembles cornmeal. Combine egg and 1 tablespoon (15 mL) of the sugar replacement. Toss with fork until well blended. Combine 1 cup (250 mL) of the crumb mixture with nuts; reserve for topping. Press remaining crumb mixture into bottom of 8-inch (20-cm) square pan coated with vegetable cooking spray. Squeeze orange; reserve ⅓ cup (80 mL) of the juice. Grind the rest of the orange (except for seeds) with cranberries. Combine reserved orange juice, water, 3 tablespoons (45 mL) of the sugar replacement, cornstarch, and allspice. Stir in cranberry–orange mixture. Cook over medium heat until thick and clear, stirring frequently. Spread over crumb crust; sprinkle with reserved nut–crumb mixture. Bake at 350° F (175° C) for 25 minutes. Cool. Cut into 2-inch (5-cm) squares.

YIELD: 16 bars
EXCHANGE 1 BAR: 1 bread, 1 fat
CALORIES 1 BAR: 92

Blueberry Muffins

1½	cups flour	375 mL
1½	teaspoons baking powder	7 mL
¼	teaspoon baking soda	1 mL
1	tablespoon canola oil	15 mL
⅓	cup egg substitute	80 mL
½	cup nonfat buttermilk	125 mL
½	teaspoon vanilla extract	2 mL
2	tablespoons nonfat sour cream	30 mL
¼	cup apple juice concentrate	60 mL
1	cup blueberries (fresh or frozen, without sugar, and defrosted)	250 mL
3	tablespoons boiling water	45 mL
2	teaspoons concentrated aspartame	10 mL

Sift together the flour, baking powder, and baking soda. Set aside. Use a wire whisk to combine the oil, egg substitute, buttermilk, vanilla extract, sour cream, and apple juice concentrate. Stir the flour mixture into the wet mixture. Do not overmix. Stir in the blueberries. Pour into a muffin tin that has been coated with nonstick cooking spray.

Bake in a preheated 375° F (190° C) oven for 30 minutes. As soon as the muffins are out of the oven, combine the boiling water and aspartame to make a glaze. Use a toothpick to make holes in the tops of the muffins. Use a pastry brush to cover the tops with the glaze.

YIELD: 12 muffins
EXCHANGE: 1 bread
CALORIES: 90

PIES

Basic Pie Shell

⅓	cup shortening	80 mL
1	cup flour	250 mL
¼	teaspoon salt	1 mL
2–4	tablespoons ice water	30–60 mL

Chill shortening. Cut shortening into flour and salt until mixture forms crumbs. Add ice water, 1 tablespoon (15 mL) at a time. Flip mixture around in bowl until a ball forms. Wrap in plastic wrap. Chill at least 1 hour. Roll to fit 9-inch (23-cm) pie pan. Fill with pie filling or prick with fork. Bake at 425° F (220° C) for 10 to 12 minutes or until firm, or leave unbaked.

YIELD: 8 servings
EXCHANGE 1 SERVING: 1 bread, 2 fat
CALORIES 1 SERVING: 170

Apple Pie Filling for Pie or Tarts

4	cups apple, peeled, sliced thin	1 L
1	tablespoon cinnamon	15 mL
1	teaspoon nutmeg	5 mL
1	tablespoon vanilla extract	15 mL
2	tablespoons lemon juice	30 mL
6	packets concentrated acesulfame-K	6 packets
1	teaspoon grated lemon peel	5 mL

Pour filling into unbaked pie or tart crust and bake as directed.

YIELD: 8 pie servings
EXCHANGE: 1 ½ fruits
CALORIES: 89

Washington's Cherry Pie

9-in.	unbaked pie shell	23-cm
2	cups unsweetened cherries	500 mL
¼	cup soft margarine	60 mL
1	tablespoon flour	15 mL
½	cup sugar replacement	125 mL
2	egg yolks	2
¼	cup evaporated milk	60 mL
½	teaspoon vanilla extract	2 mL
2	egg whites	2
2	teaspoons granulated sugar replacement	10 mL

Drain cherries; pour into unbaked pie shell. Cream margarine, flour, and sugar replacement. Add egg yolks and beat until smooth. Add evaporated milk and vanilla extract. Pour over cherries. Bake at 450° F (230° C) for 10 minutes. Reduce heat. Bake at 350° F (175° C) for 30 minutes. Whip egg whites until soft peaks form. Add granulated sugar replacement; whip until thick and stiff. Top pie filling with meringue, carefully sealing edges. Bake at 350° F (175° C) for 12 to 15 minutes, or until delicately brown.

YIELD: 8 servings
EXCHANGE 1 SERVING: 1 fruit, 1 fat, (plus pie shell exchange)
CALORIES 1 SERVING: 88
(PLUS PIE SHELL CALORIES)

Fresh Strawberry Pie

9-in.	baked pie shell	23-cm
⅝	ounce pkg. lo-cal strawberry gelatin	20-g pkg.
1	quart fresh strawberries	1 L
1	package lo-cal whipped topping (prepared)	1 package

Prepare one envelope of gelatin as directed on package. Allow to semi-set. Rinse and hull berries; place in baked pie shell. Pour gelatin over top; chill until firm. Top with prepared whipped topping.

YIELD: 8 servings
EXCHANGE 1 SERVING: ½ fruit, (PLUS PIE SHELL EXCHANGE)
CALORIES 1 SERVING: 20
(PLUS PIE SHELL CALORIES)

Fine-Crumb Pie Shell

1¼	cups fine crumbs (graham cracker, dry cereal, Zwieback)	310 mL
3	tablespoons margarine (melted)	45 mL
1	tablespoon water	15 mL
	spices (see Spices and Herbs, pages 9–10)	
	sugar replacement	

Combine crumbs with melted margarine and water; add spices and sugar replacement, if desired. Spread evenly in 9-inch (23-cm) pie pan. Press firmly onto sides and bottom. Either chill until set or bake at 325° F (165° C) for 8 to 10 minutes.

YIELD: 8 servings
EXCHANGE 1 SERVING GRAHAM CRACKER: 1 bread, 1 fat
CALORIES 1 SERVING GRAHAM CRACKER: 85
EXCHANGE 1 SERVING DRY CEREAL: ½ bread, 1 fat
CALORIES 1 SERVING DRY CEREAL: 64
EXCHANGE 1 SERVING ZWIEBACK: ½ bread, 1 fat
CALORIES 1 SERVING ZWIEBACK: 70

Blueberry Cream Pie

9-in.	baked pie shell	23-cm
2	cups lo-cal whipped topping (prepared)	500 mL
1½	cups Blueberry Topping (page 159)	375 mL

Fold prepared whipped topping into Blueberry Topping. Spread into baked pie shell. Chill until firm.

YIELD: 8 servings
EXCHANGE 1 SERVING: ½ fruit
(PLUS PIE SHELL EXCHANGE)
CALORIES 1 SERVING: 30
(PLUS PIE SHELL CALORIES)

Cranberry–Pineapple Pie

9-in.	unbaked pie shell	23-cm
1½	cups unsweetened crushed pineapple	375 mL
½	cup sugar replacement	125 mL
1	tablespoon cornstarch	15 mL
½	teaspoon salt	2 mL
1	tablespoon butter	15 mL
2	cups cranberries	500 mL

Drain pineapple; reserve liquid. Blend ½ cup (125 mL) of the pineapple liquid with cornstarch. Cook until very thick. Stir in sugar replacement, salt, and butter. Add cranberries and drained pineapple. Pour into unbaked pie shell. Bake at 425° F (220° C) for 30 to 40 minutes, or until set.

YIELD: 8 servings
EXCHANGE 1 SERVING: 1 fruit, ½ fat
(PLUS PIE SHELL EXCHANGE)
CALORIES 1 SERVING: 30
(PLUS PIE SHELL CALORIES)

Strawberry Cream Pie

9-in.	baked pie shell	23-cm
1	package lo-cal vanilla pudding	1 package
1½	cups Strawberry Topping (page 159)	375 mL
¼	cup fresh strawberries (halved)	60 mL
1	package lo-cal whipped topping (prepared)	1 package

Prepare pudding as directed on package; cool slightly. Pour into baked pie shell. Cover with waxed paper; chill until set. Combine Strawberry Topping with fresh strawberries. Spread evenly on top of pudding. Top with prepared whipped topping.

YIELD: 8 servings
EXCHANGE 1 SERVING: 1 ½ fruit, ½ milk
(PLUS PIE SHELL EXCHANGE)
CALORIES 1 SERVING: 75
(PLUS PIE SHELL CALORIES)

Lemon Cake Pie

9-in.	unbaked pie shell	23-cm
½	cup sugar replacement	125 mL
2	tablespoons flour	30 mL
2	tablespoons margarine (soft)	30 mL
1	tablespoon lemon rind	15 mL
3	tablespoons lemon juice	45 mL
1	cup skim milk	250 mL
2	eggs, separated	2

Combine sugar replacement, flour, margarine, lemon rind and juice, skim milk, and egg yolks. Beat vigorously. Fold in egg whites (well beaten). Pour into unbaked pie shell. Bake at 325° F (165° C) for 1 hour, or until set.

YIELD: 8 servings
EXCHANGE 1 SERVING: 1 milk
(PLUS PIE SHELL EXCHANGE)
CALORIES 1 SERVING: 40
(PLUS PIE SHELL CALORIES)

Fresh Rhubarb Pie

9-in.	unbaked pie shell	23-cm
1	quart 1-inch (2.5-cm) pieces rhubarb	1 L
4	tablespoons flour	60 mL
½	cup sugar replacement	125 mL
2	eggs (beaten)	2

Mix rhubarb, flour, sugar replacement, and eggs. Pour into unbaked pie shell. Bake at 350° F (175° C) for 40 to 50 minutes, or until set.

YIELD: 8 servings
EXCHANGE 1 SERVING: ½ fruit
(PLUS PIE SHELL EXCHANGE)
CALORIES 1 SERVING: 68
(PLUS PIE SHELL CALORIES)

Strawberry Turnovers

¼	teaspoon cornstarch	1 mL
1	tablespoon water	15 mL
½	cup Strawberry Topping (page 159)	125 mL
1	dough for Basic Pie Shell (page 186)	1
	Vanilla Gloss (page 222)	

Blend cornstarch and water. Add to Strawberry Topping. Cook over low heat until very thick. Roll pie dough thin. Cut into eight 4-inch (10-cm) squares. Place 1½ teaspoons (7 mL) of the strawberry mixture into center of each square. Fold each square into a triangle; press sides securely together to seal. Bake at 400° F (200° C) for 9 to 11 minutes, or until golden brown. Brush with Vanilla Gloss.

MICROWAVE: Use microwave only for strawberry filling. Blend cornstarch and water. Add to Strawberry Topping. Cook on High for 30 seconds, or until very thick. Proceed as above.

YIELD: 8 turnovers
EXCHANGE 1 TURNOVER: 1 bread
CALORIES 1 TURNOVER: 180

FRUITS

Apple-Go-Round

1	firm apple	1
¼	cup orange juice	60 mL
1	teaspoon lemon juice	5 mL
1	tablespoon raisins	15 mL
1	tablespoon celery (diced)	15 mL
2	tablespoons applesauce	30 mL
	lettuce leaf	

Slice off top of apple; remove core. Prick outside with sharp fork.
Place apple in tall narrow bowl. Combine orange and lemon juice;
pour over apple. (Add extra water if apple is not covered.) Marinate
in refrigerator 4 to 5 hours. Combine raisins, celery, and applesauce.
Allow to mellow at room temperature 2 hours. Chill thoroughly. Drain
apple. Cut apple into 8 sections, slicing almost to the bottom. Fill with
applesauce mixture. Place on crisp lettuce leaf.

YIELD: 1 serving
EXCHANGE: 2 fruit
CALORIES: 54

Baked Apple Dumpling

1	teaspoon raisins	5 mL
2	tablespoons orange juice	30 mL
½	teaspoon sugar replacement	2 mL
1	small apple	1 small
	biscuit dough for 1 biscuit	

Combine raisins and orange juice in saucepan. Heat to a boil. Add sugar replacement. Cover. Allow to rest while preparing remaining ingredients. Core apple; with a fork or toothpick, prick the inside of the apple cavity. On floured board, roll biscuit dough very thin and large enough to wrap around apple. Place apple in center of dough. Fill apple cavity with raisin mixture. Wrap dough around apple and secure at top. Place in baking dish. Bake at 375° F (190° C) for 25 to 30 minutes.

YIELD: 1 serving
EXCHANGE: 1 bread, 1 fruit
CALORIES: 142

Sweet 'n' Sour Strawberries

2	cups fresh or frozen strawberries with no sugar added	500 mL
3	packets concentrated acesulfame-K	3 packets
2	tablespoons balsamic vinegar	30 mL

Slice the strawberries in half. Sprinkle them with acesulfame-K and vinegar. Stir to combine. This is best served chilled, and is a real "company" dessert when presented in fancy glasses.

YIELD: 4 servings
EXCHANGE: ⅓ fruit
CALORIES: 24

Apple Crisp

4	cups apples, sliced	1 L
¼	cup water	60 mL
1	tablespoon molasses	15 mL
3	packets concentrated acesulfame-K	3 packets
1	tablespoon lemon juice	15 mL
1	teaspoon cinnamon	5 mL
¼	teaspoon cloves	1 mL
¾	cup oatmeal	185 mL
2	teaspoons margarine or butter	10 mL
2	packets concentrated acesulfame-K	2 packets

Combine the apples, water, molasses, 3 packets of acesulfame-K, lemon juice, cinnamon, and cloves. Mix well. Arrange the apple mixture in an 8-inch (20-cm) square baking dish coated with nonstick cooking spray. Combine the remaining ingredients and sprinkle the mixture over the apples. Bake at 375° F (190° C) for 30 minutes or until the apples are tender and the topping is lightly browned.

YIELD: 8 servings
EXCHANGE: 1 bread
CALORIES: 84

Peach Melba

½	cup raspberries	125 mL
½	teaspoon sugar replacement	2 mL
½	cup dietetic vanilla ice cream	125 mL
½	peach (sliced)	½

Slightly mash raspberries and sugar replacement. Allow to rest 5 minutes. Place ice cream in dish. Top with peach slices and raspberries.

YIELD: 1 serving
EXCHANGE: 1 bread, 1 fruit, 1 fat
CALORIES: 120

Nectarine Purée

3	fresh, sweet nectarines	3
2	teaspoons lemon juice	10 mL
2	teaspoons concentrated aspartame	10 mL

Drop the nectarines into a large pan of boiling water. Turn off the heat. Let stand for one minute to loosen the skins. Drain the hot water, then pour cold water over the fruit and slip off their skins. Place the nectarines in a food processor or blender with the lemon juice and aspartame. The amount of aspartame will vary, depending on the tartness of the fruit. Purée. Spoon into glass dessert dishes.

YIELD: 3 servings
EXCHANGE: 1 fruit
CALORIES: 68

Browned Bananas

1	banana, peeled	1

Slice the banana in half lengthwise. Place it on a broiler pan that has been coated with nonstick cooking spray. Place the pan under a preheated broiler a few inches from the heat. Watch it carefully and remove the tray from the oven as the banana becomes browned and bubbly. Serve hot. A small dollop of sugar-free, frozen nonfat vanilla yogurt makes a nice garnish for this dessert.

YIELD: 2 servings
EXCHANGE: 1 fruit
CALORIES: 53

Poached Pears and Raspberries

6	medium pears	6
1	packet concentrated acesulfame-K (or 1 tablespoon sugar/15 mL)	1 packet
¼	cup water	60 mL
1-in.	piece of vanilla bean, slit	2.5 cm
2	cups raspberries, fresh or frozen, unsweetened	500 mL
2	tablespoons fruit-only, seedless raspberry jam	30 mL

Peel, core, and halve the pears. Combine the acesulfame (or sugar) and water in a saucepan and bring to a boil. Reduce the heat to low and add the vanilla bean and pear halves. Cover. Simmer for 5 minutes or so, until the pears are fork-tender. Cool. Drain. In a small bowl, gently toss the raspberries and jam. Put two pear halves on each serving plate. Mound the raspberries on top of the pears.

YIELD: 6 servings
EXCHANGE: 2 fruits
CALORIES: 168

Four-Fruit Compote

1	large orange	1
1	small cantaloupe	1
½	pound seedless grapes	250 g
3	ripe pears	3
½	cup water	125 mL
3	tablespoons lemon juice	45 mL
3	packets concentrated acesulfame-K	3 packets
¼	teaspoon mace	1 mL
2	tablespoons rum (optional)	30 mL

Cut the orange into segments, remove the membrane, and put the segments into a large bowl. Peel the cantaloupe, cut it crosswise, and remove the seeds. Cut into large cubes. Add the cubes and the stemmed grapes to the oranges. Core the pears, then cut them into large cubes. Sprinkle the pear cubes with lemon juice and add them to the fruit bowl. Mix together the water, lemon juice, acesulfame-K, and mace. Add rum, if desired. Cover; refrigerate for an hour or more before serving.

YIELD: 8 servings
EXCHANGE: 1 fruit
CALORIES: 76

Mixed-Berry Smoothie

12-ounce can evaporated nonfat milk		354-mL can
1	tablespoon cornstarch	15 mL
3	packets concentrated acesulfame-K	3 packets
1	teaspoon almond extract	5 mL
1	teaspoon concentrated aspartame	5 mL
12-ounce bag frozen mixed berries		340-g bag
2	cups nonfat yogurt, no sugar added (plain or vanilla)	500 mL

Combine the first three ingredients and stir them together in a saucepan. Heat just to a boil, then reduce the heat and simmer for 5 minutes or until the sauce thickens; stir constantly with a wire whisk. Turn off the heat, stirring in the almond extract, aspartame, and berries. Let cool and then fold in the yogurt.

YIELD: 8 servings
EXCHANGE: 1 milk
CALORIES: 99

Ambrosia

2	oranges, peeled with membranes removed	2
2	teaspoons measures-like-sugar aspartame	10 mL
2	bananas, peeled	2
¼	cup shredded coconut	60 mL

Slice the oranges and bananas thin. Place a layer of orange slices in the bottom of a serving bowl. Sprinkle with some of the aspartame. Place a layer of bananas over the oranges, then a layer of coconut. Make many layers of fruit, ending with a layer of coconut. Cover with plastic wrap; refrigerate for at least an hour before serving.

YIELD: 4 servings
EXCHANGE: 1½ fruit, ½ fat
CALORIES: 84

PUDDINGS, CUSTARDS, AND GELATINS

Rhubarb Pudding

1	quart rhubarb (cut in pieces)	1 L
1	cup water	250 mL
2	tablespoons cornstarch	30 mL
1	teaspoon sugar replacement	5 mL

Cut rhubarb into pieces. Place rhubarb in saucepan. Add the water. Cook rhubarb until tender. Mix cornstarch with small amount of cold water; add to rhubarb. Cook until thickened. Remove from heat; add sugar replacement. Stir until dissolved.

MICROWAVE: Place rhubarb in large bowl. Add the water. Cook on High for 4 minutes, or until tender. Mix cornstarch with small amount of cold water; add to rhubarb. Cook on High for 1 to 2 minutes, or until thickened.

YIELD: 6 servings
EXCHANGE 1 SERVING: ⅛ fruit, ⅛ bread
CALORIES 1 SERVING: 22

Raisin Rice Pudding

1	package lo-cal rice pudding	1 package
½	cup raisins	125 mL

Prepare rice pudding as directed on package. Soak raisins in warm water for 1 hour. Drain thoroughly. Add raisins to rice pudding.

YIELD: 5 servings, ½ cup (125 mL) each
EXCHANGE 1 SERVING: ½ bread, ½ milk, ½ fruit
CALORIES 1 SERVING: 100

Bread Pudding

½	loaf "light" sourdough bread	½ loaf
	12-ounce can evaporated skim milk	375-mL can
½	cup unsweetened applesauce	125 mL
1	teaspoon vanilla extract	5 mL
½	cup skim milk	125 mL
8	packets acesulfame-K	8 packets
⅓	cup raisins	80 mL
½	teaspoon cinnamon	2 mL
4	egg whites	4

Cut the bread slices into cubes; place them on a cookie sheet coated with nonstick cooking spray. Place the tray in a preheated 350° F (175° C) oven for 10 minutes. Combine all the other ingredients and add the bread. Toss well and place in an ovenproof baking dish that has been sprayed with nonstick vegetable cooking spray. Place this baking dish in a large pan of water filled nearly to the top of the baking dish, and place the pan in a preheated 350° F (175° C) oven. Bake for 40 minutes. Serve hot or cold.

YIELD: 8 servings
EXCHANGE: 1 ½ bread
CALORIES: 109

Baked Custard

12-ounce can evaporated skim milk		375-mL can
2	packets acesulfame-K	2 packets
1	teaspoon sugar	5 mL
1	teaspoon lemon peel	5 mL
1	teaspoon margarine or butter	5 mL
¼	cup egg substitute	60 mL
1	teaspoon vanilla extract	5 mL
	sprinkling nutmeg (optional)	

Heat the milk over hot water in the top of a double boiler. Add the acesulfame-K, sugar, lemon peel, and margarine and whisk together for a few minutes. In a separate bowl, use an electric mixer to beat the egg substitute for a few minutes until foamy and light. Add a little hot milk mixture to the beaten egg substitute and beat. Gradually pour in the rest of the hot milk and beat constantly. Add the vanilla extract and heat briefly. Pour into small ovenproof custard dishes that have been coated with nonstick cooking spray. If desired, sprinkle the top with nutmeg. Place the small cups in a larger pan of hot water. Bake in a preheated 325° F (165° C) oven for approximately 40 minutes. A knife inserted in the center should come out clean. Chill before serving.

YIELD: 4 servings
EXCHANGE: 1 milk
CALORIES: 97

Tapioca Pudding

3	cups skim milk	750 mL
¼	cup quick-cooking (instant) tapioca	60 mL
¼	teaspoon salt (optional)	1 mL
¼	cup egg substitute	60 mL
1	egg white, beaten	1
1	teaspoon vanilla extract	5 mL

| 2½ | teaspoons concentrated aspartame | 12 mL |

Whisk together the milk, tapioca, salt (optional), egg substitute, and beaten egg white in the top of a double boiler. Heat the water in the lower part to boiling. Cover the top part and cook for five minutes while stirring. Remove from the heat; add the vanilla extract and aspartame. The pudding will thicken as it cools.

YIELD: 6 servings
EXCHANGE: 1 bread, ½ milk
CALORIES: 79

Pineapple Mousse

	20-ounce can pineapple, packed in juice, drained	625-mL can
2	tablespoons fructose	30 mL
1	cup evaporated skim milk, chilled	250 mL
1	envelope unflavored gelatin	1 envelope
1	tablespoon lemon juice	15 mL

Purée the pineapple in a blender or food processor. Add the fructose; stir. Set aside. In a mixing bowl, whip the evaporated milk until thick and creamy. In the top of a double boiler, sprinkle the gelatin over the lemon juice. Let stand 3 to 5 minutes. Stir over hot water until dissolved. Stir the gelatin into the whipped milk. Fold the pineapple mixture into the milk. Spoon into dessert dishes. Chill until set.

YIELD: 16 servings
EXCHANGE: ⅛ milk, ⅛ fruit
CALORIES: 51

Chocolate Pudding

¼	cup sugar	60 mL
3	packets concentrated acesulfame-K	3 packets
2	tablespoons unsweetened cocoa powder	30 mL
3	tablespoons cornstarch	45 mL
2	cups nonfat milk	500 mL
1	teaspoon vanilla extract	5 mL

Combine the sugar, acesulfame-K, cocoa, and cornstarch in a saucepan. Add about ½ cup (125 mL) milk. Stir with a wire whisk until dissolved and the mixture is smooth. Add the remaining milk and vanilla extract. Cook, stirring occasionally until thick, about 5 minutes. Cool before serving.

YIELD: 4 servings
EXCHANGE: 1 bread, ½ milk
CALORIES: 118

Lemon Pudding

1	envelope unflavored gelatin, unsweetened	1 envelope
2	tablespoons cold water	30 mL
½	cup boiling water	125 mL
1½	cups nonfat buttermilk	375 mL
2	teaspoons lemon rind	10 mL
2	teaspoons lemon juice	10 mL
2	teaspoons concentrated aspartame	10 mL
2	drops yellow food coloring (optional)	2 drops

In a large mixing bowl, sprinkle the gelatin over the cold water to soften. Let sit for a few minutes. Pour the boiling water over it and stir until completely dissolved. Add the remaining ingredients and whisk together. Pour into five individual pudding dishes that have been sprayed very lightly with nonstick cooking spray. The pudding may be served in the individual dishes or unmolded onto separate plates. This pudding can be served plain or dressed up with a little fresh fruit or a plain, frozen strawberry.

YIELD: 5 servings
EXCHANGE: ½ milk
CALORIES: 31

Black Cherry Gelatin

1	envelope flavored gelatin	1 envelope
¼	cup cold water	60 mL
2	packets concentrated acesulfame-K	2 packets
2	cups sugar-free black cherry soda	500 mL

Sprinkle the gelatin over the water in the top of a double boiler. Let stand for 5 minutes. Meanwhile, in another bowl, combine the remaining ingredients. Stir the gelatin over hot water until dissolved. Pour into the black cherry mixture. Chill until set. Garnish with fresh fruit slices if desired.

YIELD: 4 servings
EXCHANGE: negligible
CALORIES: 7

Jell Jells

1	quart lo-cal orange soda	1 L
4	envelopes unflavored gelatin	4 envelopes
1½	packages lo-cal orange gelatin	1½ packages

Bring orange soda to a boil. Combine gelatins together in large bowl; add boiling soda. Stir to dissolve. Pour into a pan. Chill until firm. Cut into cubes.

EXCHANGE: Negligible
CALORIES: Negligible

Homemade Ice Cream

	13-ounce can evaporated milk	385-mL can
2	tablespoons sugar replacement	30 mL
1½	cups whole milk	375 mL
1	tablespoon vanilla extract	15 mL
3	eggs (well beaten)	3

Combine evaporated milk and sugar replacement. Beat well until sugar is dissolved. Add whole milk and vanilla extract; beat well. Add eggs; beat eggs into milk mixture vigorously. Pour into ice cream maker. Freeze according to manufacturer's directions.

YIELD: 8 servings
EXCHANGE 1 SERVING: ½ milk, ½ lean meat
CALORIES 1 SERVING: 122

Lemon Ice Freeze

1	envelope unflavored gelatin	1 envelope
1½	cups milk	375 mL
2	egg yolks (slightly beaten)	2
¼	teaspoon salt	1 mL
½	cup sugar replacement	125 mL
2	teaspoons lemon extract	10 mL
2	tablespoons lemon peel	30 mL
2	egg whites (stiffly beaten)	2

Soften gelatin in ¼ cup (60 mL) of the milk; set aside. Combine egg yolks, remaining milk, salt, sugar replacement, lemon extract, and peel in top of double boiler. Cook until thick and creamy. Remove from heat. Add gelatin mixture; stir until dissolved. Cool. Pour into ice cube tray and freeze. Place mixture in cold bowl and beat until smooth; fold in stiffly beaten egg whites. Return to tray and refreeze.

YIELD: 6 servings
EXCHANGE 1 SERVING: ½ milk, ⅓ meat
CALORIES 1 SERVING: 100

Frozen Strawberry Yogurt

1	8-ounce pkg. frozen strawberries, no sugar added	1 226-g pkg.
1½	teaspoons lemon juice	7 mL
2	teaspoons aspartame	10 mL
1	tablespoon vanilla extract	15 mL
1½	cups nonfat yogurt, no sugar added (plain or vanilla)	375 mL

Put fruit in food processor with flavorings. Purée; add yogurt. Freeze in small yogurt containers for easy serving.

YIELD: 6 servings
EXCHANGE: ⅓ milk
CALORIES: 76

Banana Sherbet

1	cup nonfat, sugar-free, banana-cream-pie–flavored yogurt	250 mL
1	cup mashed bananas	250 mL
1	teaspoon concentrated aspartame	5 mL
1	teaspoon vanilla extract	5 mL
½	teaspoon banana extract	2 mL

Combine all the ingredients in a food processor. Pour into two small yogurt containers; freeze for a few hours or overnight.

YIELD: 4 servings
EXCHANGE: 1 fruit, ½ milk
CALORIES: 104

Frosty Frozen Dessert

1	egg white	1
⅓	cup water	80 mL
⅓	cup nonfat dry milk	80 mL
⅓	cup egg substitute	80 mL
⅓	cup measures-like-sugar aspartame	80 mL
¾	cup fruit purée such as nectarines	185 mL

Use an electric mixer to beat together the first three ingredients until a stiff mixture forms. Set aside. Take a separate mixing bowl and beat together the remaining ingredients until smooth. Put the bowl of beaten egg white back under the beaters, then gently beat the fruit-and-egg-substitute mixture into the beaten egg white. Pour into small yogurt containers and freeze for several hours or overnight.

YIELD: 11 servings, ½ cup (125 mL) each
EXCHANGE: ½ milk
CALORIES: 36

Icy Grapes

Wash grapes and place them in the freezer for several hours or overnight. Serve in fancy wine glasses.

YIELD: 1 serving, ½ cup (125 mL)
EXCHANGE: 1 fruit
CALORIES: 54

DESSERTS FOR SPECIAL OCCASIONS

Grand Marnier Soufflé for Six

2	tablespoons margarine or butter	30 mL
2½	tablespoons regular all-purpose flour	37 mL
¾	cup skim milk	185 mL
1	packet concentrated acesulfame-K	1 packet
2	egg yolks, beaten	2
3	egg whites	3
⅛	teaspoon cream of tartar	½ mL
3	tablespoons Grand Marnier	45 mL

In a saucepan, melt the margarine or butter and remove it from the heat. Stir in the flour and milk; cook, stirring over medium heat, until thickened and smooth. Stir in the acesulfame-K; cool slightly; add egg yolks.

In a medium bowl, beat the egg whites until foamy; add the cream of tartar, beating until stiff peaks form when the beater is raised. Gently fold the egg yolk mixture and Grand Marnier into the egg whites. Turn into a 1-quart (1-L) soufflé dish or casserole coated with nonstick cooking spray. Bake for 10 minutes in a preheated 450° F (230° C) oven, then turn down the heat to 325° F (165° C) and bake 15 minutes longer. Serve immediately.

YIELD: 6 servings
EXCHANGE: 1 fat, 1 bread
CALORIES: 122

Hot Apple Soufflé

½	cup margarine or butter	125 mL
½	cup flour	125 mL
2	cups cold skim milk	500 mL
2	tablespoons granulated sugar	30 mL
1	packet concentrated acesulfame-K	1 packet
	grated peel from ½ lemon	
2	medium apples	2
4	eggs, separated	4
2	tablespoons slivered toasted almonds	30 mL

About 2¼ hours before serving, melt the margarine in a medium saucepan; stir in the flour, then the milk. Cook, stirring constantly, until smooth and thickened. Blend in the sugar, acesulfame-K, and lemon peel; let cool slightly, stirring occasionally.

Meanwhile, wash, pare, and core the apples, then cut each into about 10 lengthwise wedges. Arrange them evenly over the bottom of a 2-quart (2 L) casserole. Beat the egg whites until stiff. Blend the yolks into the flour–milk mixture, then carefully fold in the egg whites. Pour this mixture over the apples, then sprinkle it with almonds. Bake in a preheated 325° F (165° C) oven for 1¼ hours or until light brown and firm. Serve at once.

YIELD: 8 servings
EXCHANGE: 1 bread, ½ meat, 1 fat
CALORIES: 229

Chocolate Soufflé

½	cup unsweetened cocoa powder	125 mL
2	tablespoons powdered sugar	30 mL
½	cup measures-like-sugar saccharin	125 mL
7	packets concentrated acesulfame-K	7 packets
2	tablespoons cornstarch	30 mL
	dash salt (optional)	
½	cup nonfat milk	125 mL
½	cup water	125 mL
4	egg whites	4
½	teaspoon cream of tartar	2 mL
¼	cup egg substitute	60 mL
1	teaspoon vanilla extract	5 mL
2	tablespoons measures-like-sugar aspartame	30 mL

Sift the cocoa, sugar, saccharin, acesulfame-K, salt, and cornstarch together twice. Put them in the top of a double boiler and add the nonfat milk and water. Whisk constantly while cooking until the mixture is smooth and thick, about eight minutes. Remove from the heat. Beat the egg whites with an electric mixer until they hold their shape; add the cream of tartar and continue beating until stiff peaks form. Pour the egg substitute and vanilla extract into the chocolate mixture. Mix. Add a small amount of the beaten egg whites into the chocolate mixture to lighten. Then use a rubber spatula to fold in the rest of the egg whites.

Pour into a 6 cup (1.5 L) soufflé dish that has been coated with nonstick cooking spray. Bake in a preheated 400° F (200° C) oven for 20 minutes. Do not overcook; the center will be a little runny to make a sauce. As soon as the soufflé is out of the oven, dust aspartame over the top.

YIELD: 8 servings
EXCHANGE: ½ bread
CALORIES: 54

Fruit Trifle

Trifles are usually served in large, straight-sided, clear-glass pedestal bowls. A traditional trifle consists of layers of brandy-soaked cake, fruit, pudding, and whipped cream. Trifles look beautiful and are delicious. When you're serving a crowd, a trifle is sure to please.

To assemble a trifle, use angel food cake, hot-milk sponge cake, or yellow cake. Tear the cake into 2 x 2-inch (5 x 5-cm) bits and spread some on the bottom of the trifle bowl. Drop on a layer of sugar-free vanilla pudding, then add a layer of fruit. Blueberries, kiwis, and strawberries make an attractive and delicious combination. Then add a layer of sugar-free whipped topping. After the topping layer, start again with cake. Make as many layers as you have ingredients and room in the dish. Or, make individual trifles with pudding, fruit, topping, and a bit of leftover cake. Assemble the layers in wine or champagne glasses for a festive look.

Here are a few tips to make trifles suitable for people on diabetic diets:

- Most "low-sugar/low-fat" whipped toppings dissolve after half an hour or so. That means you need to assemble the trifle close to serving time.

- Use only ingredients that you know are suitable. Stay away from frozen or canned puddings or fruit with sugar.

- Bananas need to be tossed in lemon juice if you're using banana slices. Otherwise, they turn dark, gooey, and unappetizing.

- Traditional trifle recipes call for cake soaked in brandy or other liqueur. We leave that out and instead add brandy extract to the pudding.

Cream Puffs

The Puff Pastry

1	cup water	250 mL
⅓	cup canola oil	80 mL
1	cup flour	250 mL
4	eggs or equivalent egg substitute	4
1	teaspoon butter-flavored extract	5 mL

Heat the water and oil to a rolling boil. Lower the heat and add the flour all at once, stirring with a wooden spoon until mixture forms a ball. Remove from the heat. With an electric mixer, beat in the eggs thoroughly, one at a time. Add the butter-flavored extract. Using a spoon, drop 12 cream puffs onto ungreased cookie sheets. Bake in a 400° F (200° C) oven for 10 minutes. Reduce the heat to 350° F (175° C) and bake for 25 minutes longer. Do not remove the cream puffs from the oven until they are quite firm to the touch. Cool the shells away from drafts before filling. To fill, cut horizontally using a sharp knife. If any damp dough remains inside, scoop it out before filling.

Fill the shells with pudding. Top with whipped topping and Chocolate Topping (page 222).

YIELD: 12 cream puffs
EXCHANGE: ½ bread, ⅓ medium-fat meat, 1 fat
CALORIES: 101

Crepes

This recipe makes fourteen 5-inch (12.5-cm) crepes. You can make them in a larger skillet and use Strawberry or Blueberry Topping (page 159) or a different fruit filling such as fruit-only jam.

1	packet concentrated acesulfame-K	1 packet
1	cup skim milk	250 mL
2	tablespoons safflower oil	30 mL
½	cup egg substitute	125 mL
½	cup flour	125 mL
2	teaspoons baking powder	10 mL
¼	teaspoon vanilla extract	1 mL

Combine all the ingredients in a blender and blend for a minute or so, or mix with an electric mixer until the batter is smooth. Heat a small, oiled skillet or crepe pan until a drop of water "dances" when you splash it on the hot surface. Add ⅓ cup (80 mL) of the batter and move the pan around so the batter covers evenly. Cook over medium heat on one side until the edges are browned and there are bubbles throughout the crepe. Turn and cook on the other side to brown. Spoon 1 tablespoon (15 mL) of Strawberry Topping or other filling on each crepe and roll the crepes up. Top with a dollop of your favorite whipped topping.

YIELD: 14 crepes, 5 inches (12.5 cm)
EXCHANGE: ½ fat
CALORIES: 44
(PLUS CALORIES AND EXCHANGES FOR FILLING AND TOPPING)

Crepes Suzette Sauce

¾	cup orange juice	185 mL
1	teaspoon grated orange peel	5 mL
1½	teaspoons cornstarch	7 mL
1	packet concentrated acesulfame-K	1 packet
1	teaspoon margarine or butter	5 mL
1	teaspoon concentrated aspartame	5 mL
½	teaspoon orange extract (use 1 teaspoon [5 mL] if liqueur is omitted)	2 mL
2	tablespoons orange-flavored liqueur, such as Grand Marnier	30 mL

In a saucepan, whisk together the orange juice, orange peel, cornstarch, and acesulfame-K. Heat to boiling, then immediately reduce the heat and cook over a medium flame, stirring constantly. When the mixture is thickened, turn off the heat.

Stir in the margarine, aspartame, orange extract, and liqueur, if desired. Take each crepe and fold in half, then again, and arrange on a separate plate. Spoon a little Crepes Suzette Sauce over each.

YIELD: 6 servings
EXCHANGE: Negligible
CALORIES: 22

CANDY

Fudge Candy

13-ounce can evaporated milk		385-mL can
3	tablespoons cocoa	45 mL
¼	cup butter	60 mL
1	tablespoon sugar replacement	15 mL
	dash salt	
1	teaspoon vanilla extract	5 mL
2½	cups unsweetened cereal crumbs	625 mL
¼	cup nuts (very finely chopped)	60 mL

Combine milk and cocoa in saucepan; cook and beat over low heat until cocoa is dissolved. Add butter, sugar replacement, salt, and vanilla. Bring to a boil; reduce heat and cook for 2 minutes. Remove from heat; add cereal crumbs and work in with wooden spoon. Cool 15 minutes. Divide in half; roll each half into a tube, 8 inches (20 cm) long. Roll each tube in finely chopped nuts. Wrap in waxed paper; chill overnight. Cut into ¼-inch (6-mm) slices.

YIELD: 64 slices
EXCHANGE 2 SLICES: ½ bread, ½ fat
CALORIES 2 SLICES: 60

Chocolate Butter Creams

1	3-ounce pkg. cream cheese (softened)	90-g pkg.
2	tablespoons skim milk	30 mL
1½	teaspoons white vanilla extract	7 mL
1	cup powdered sugar replacement	250 mL
1	recipe Chocolate Topping (page 222)	1 recipe

Beat cream cheese, milk, and vanilla until fluffy; stir in powdered sugar replacement. Form into 30 balls and dip each one in chocolate.

YIELD: 30 creams
EXCHANGE 1 CREAM: ¼ low-fat milk
CALORIES 1 CREAM: 31

Chocolate Crunch Candy

1	cup nonfat dry milk powder	250 mL
½	cup cocoa	125 mL
2	tablespoons liquid fructose	30 mL
3	tablespoons water	45 mL
1½	cups chow mein noodles	375 mL

Combine milk powder and cocoa in food processor or blender, blending to a fine powder. Stir in fructose and water and beat until smooth and creamy. Slightly crush the chow mein noodles and fold them into chocolate mixture. Drop by teaspoonfuls onto waxed paper. Cool at room temperature.

YIELD: 30 pieces
EXCHANGE 1 PIECE: ⅕ bread
CALORIES 1 PIECE: 11

Butter Sticks

7	large shredded wheat biscuits	7 large
½	cup crunchy peanut butter	125 mL
3	tablespoons granulated sugar replacement	45 mL
2	egg whites	2
1	tablespoon flour	15 mL
1	tablespoon water	15 mL
1	tablespoon baking powder	15 mL
1	teaspoon vanilla extract	5 mL
1	recipe Chocolate Topping (page 222)	1 recipe

Break biscuits into large bowl or food processor. Add peanut butter, sugar replacement, egg whites, flour, water, baking powder, and vanilla. Work with wooden spoon or steel blade until mixture is completely blended; mixture will be sticky. Form into 16 sticks and place them on an ungreased cookie sheet. Bake at 400° F (200° C) for 10 minutes, or until surface feels hard. Remove; cool slightly. Dip in chocolate.

YIELD: 16 sticks
EXCHANGE 1 STICK: ⅓ bread, 1 fat
CALORIES 1 STICK: 115

Sugared Pecans

½	cup water	125 mL
¼	cup granulated sugar replacement	60 mL
¼	cup granulated brown sugar replacement	60 mL
1	cup pecan halves	250 mL

Combine water and sugar replacements in saucepan, stirring to dissolve. Bring to boil, and boil for 3 minutes. Stir in pecans until completely coated; remove pan from heat. Allow pecans to rest in sugar water for 2 to 3 minutes. Remove with slotted spoon and cool completely.

YIELD: 1 cup (250 mL)
EXCHANGE ⅒ OF CUP: 1 fat
CALORIES ⅒ OF CUP: 48

Cookie Brittle

½	cup margarine	125 mL
2	teaspoons vanilla extract	10 mL
1	teaspoon salt	5 mL
3	tablespoons granulated sugar replacement	45 mL
2	cups flour (sifted)	500 mL
1	cup semisweet chocolate chips	250 mL
½	cup walnuts (chopped fine)	125 mL

Combine margarine, vanilla, salt, and sugar replacement in mixing bowl or food processor; beat until smooth. Stir in flour, chocolate chips, and walnuts. Press into ungreased 15 x 10-inch (39 x 25-cm) pan. Bake at 375° F (190° C) for 25 minutes. Remove from oven, score into 2 x 1-inch (5 x 2.5-cm) pieces and cool completely. Break into candy pieces.

YIELD: 60 pieces
EXCHANGE 1 PIECE: ½ fat, ⅓ bread
CALORIES 1 PIECE: 48

Fruit Candy Bars

1	envelope unflavored gelatin	1 envelope
¼	cup water	60 mL
1	cup dried apricots	250 mL
1	cup raisins	250 mL

1	cup pecans	250 mL
1	tablespoon flour	15 mL
2	tablespoons orange peel (grated)	30 mL
1	teaspoon rum extract	5 mL

Sprinkle gelatin over water in a saucepan; allow to soften for 5 minutes. Heat and stir until gelatin is completely dissolved. Combine apricots, raisins, pecans, flour, and orange peel in blender or food processor, working until finely chopped. Add to gelatin mixture. Add rum extract and stir to completely blend. Line 8-inch (20-cm) square pan with plastic wrap or waxed paper. Spread fruit mixture evenly into pan, and set aside to cool completely until candy is firm. Turn out onto cutting board, cut into 24 bars and wrap individually.

YIELD: 24 bars
EXCHANGE 1 BAR: 1 fruit, ½ fat
CALORIES 1 BAR: 68

Coconut Macaroons

1	cup evaporated skim milk	250 mL
2	teaspoons granulated sugar replacement	10 mL
3	cups unsweetened coconut (shredded)	750 mL

Combine milk and sugar replacement in large bowl, stirring until sugar replacement dissolves. Add coconut and stir until coconut is completely moistened. Drop by teaspoonfuls onto greased cookie sheets, 2 to 3 inches (5 to 7.5 cm) apart. Bake at 350° F (175° C) for 15 minutes, or until tops are lightly browned. Remove from pan immediately.

YIELD: 48 drops
EXCHANGE 1 DROP: ½ fat
CALORIES 1 DROP: 31

Chocolate Topping

3	cups skim milk	750 mL
2	ounces unsweetened chocolate	60 g
3	tablespoons cornstarch	45 mL
½	cup sugar replacement	125 mL
1	teaspoon salt	5 mL
2	tablespoons butter	30 mL
2	teaspoons vanilla extract	10 mL

Combine skim milk, chocolate, cornstarch, sugar replacement, and salt in saucepan. Bring to a full boil. Boil for 2 to 3 minutes; remove from heat. Add butter and vanilla extract.

YIELD: 3 cups (750 mL)
EXCHANGE 2 TABLESPOONS (30 mL): ⅛ milk
CALORIES 2 TABLESPOONS (30 mL): 35

Vanilla Gloss

¼	cup cold water	60 mL
2	teaspoons cornstarch	10 mL
	dash salt	
⅓	cup sugar replacement	80 mL
1	teaspoon vanilla extract	5 mL

Blend cold water and cornstarch. Pour into small saucepan. Add salt. Boil until clear and thickened. Remove from heat. Add sugar replacement and vanilla extract. Stir to dissolve. Cool.

YIELD: ¼ cup (60 mL)
EXCHANGE: Negligible
CALORIES: Negligible

FOOD EXCHANGE LISTS

ONE STARCH EXCHANGE EQUALS

15 grams carbohydrate,
0–3 grams protein,
0–1 grams fat, and
80 calories.

BREAD	SERVING SIZE
Bagel, large (about 4 oz)	¼ (1 oz)
Biscuit, 2½ inches across	1
Bread, reduced-calorie	2 slices (1½ oz)
Bread, white, whole-grain, pumpernickel, rye, unfrosted raisin	1 slice (1 oz)
Bread sticks, crisp, 4 inches long x ½ inch	2 (⅔ oz)
Chapatti, small, 6 inches across	1
Cornbread, 1¾ inch cube	1 (1½ oz)
English muffin	½
Hot dog or hamburger bun	½ (1 oz)
Naan, 8 inches by 2 inches	¼
Pancake, 4 inches across, ¼ inch thick	1
Pita, 6 inches across	½
Roll, plain, small	1 (1 oz)
Stuffing, bread	⅓ cup
Taco shell, 5 inches across	2
Tortilla, corn, 6 inches across	1
Tortilla, flour, 6 inches across	1
Tortilla, flour, 10 inches across	⅓ tortilla
Waffle, 4-inch square or 4 inches across	1

CEREALS AND GRAINS	SERVING SIZE
Barley, cooked	⅓ cup
Bran, dry	
oat	¼ cup
wheat	½ cup
Bulgur (cooked)	½ cup
Cereals	
bran	½ cup
cooked (oats, oatmeal)	½ cup
puffed	1½ cups
shredded wheat, plain	½ cup
sugar-coated	½ cup
unsweetened, ready-to-eat	¾ cup
Cornmeal (dry)	3 Tbsp

ONE STARCH EXCHANGE EQUALS

15 grams carbohydrate,
0–3 grams protein,
0–1 grams fat, and
80 calories.

CEREALS AND GRAINS	SERVING SIZE
Couscous	⅓ cup
Flour (dry)	3 Tbsp
Granola, low-fat	¼ cup
Grape-Nuts	¼ cup
Grits, cooked	½ cup
Kasha	½ cup
Millet, cooked	⅓ cup
Muesli	¼ cup
Oats	½ cup
Pasta, cooked	⅓ cup
Polenta, cooked	⅓ cup
Quinoa, cooked	⅓ cup
Rice, white or brown, cooked	⅓ cup
Rice milk	½ cup
Tabbouleh (tabouli), prepared	½ cup
Wheat germ	3 Tbsp
Wild rice, cooked	½ cup

STARCHY VEGETABLES	SERVING SIZE
Cassava	⅓ cup
Corn	½ cup
Corn on cob, large	½ cob (5 oz)
Hominy, canned	¾ cup
Mixed vegetables with corn, peas, or pasta	1 cup
Parsnips	½ cup
Peas, green	½ cup
Plantain, ripe	⅓ cup
Potato	
baked with skin	¼ large (3 oz)
boiled, all kinds	½ cup or ½
mashed, with milk and fat	½ cup
French fried (oven-baked)	1 cup (2 oz)
Pumpkin, canned, no sugar added	1 cup
Spaghetti/pasta sauce	½ cup
Squash, winter (acorn, butternut, pumpkin)	1 cup
Succotash	½ cup
Yam, sweet potato, plain	½ cup

ONE STARCH EXCHANGE EQUALS

15 grams carbohydrate,
0–3 grams protein,
0–1 grams fat, and
80 calories.

CRACKERS AND SNACKS	SERVING SIZE
Animal crackers	8
Crackers	
round-butter type	6
saltine-type	6
sandwich-style, cheese or peanut butter filling	3
whole-wheat regular	2–5 (¾ oz)
whole-wheat lower fat or crispbreads	2–5 (¾ oz)
Graham crackers, 2½ inch square	3
Matzoh	¾ oz
Melba toast, about 2-inch by 4-inch piece	4 pieces
Oyster crackers	20
Popcorn	3 cups
with butter	3 cups
no fat added	3 cups
lower fat	3 cups
Pretzels	¾ oz
Rice cakes, 4 inches across	2
Snack chips	
fat-free or baked (tortilla, potato), baked pita chips	15–20 (¾ oz)
regular (tortilla, potato)	9–13 (¾ oz)

BEANS, PEAS, AND LENTILS	SERVING SIZE

(Count as 1 starch exchange, plus 1 lean meat exchange.)

Baked beans	⅓ cup
Beans and peas (black, black-eyed, garbanzo, kidney, lima, navy, pinto, split, white)	½ cup
Lentils, cooked (brown, green, yellow)	½ cup
Miso*	3 Tbsp
Refried beans, canned	½ cup

*= 400 mg or more sodium per exchange

STARCHY FOODS PREPARED WITH FAT	SERVING SIZE

(Count as 1 starch exchange, plus 1 fat exchange.)

Biscuit, 2½ inches across	1
Chow mein noodles	½ cup
Corn bread, 2 inch cube	1 (2 oz)
Crackers, round butter type	6
Croutons	1 cup
French-fried potatoes	16–25 (3 oz)
Granola	¼ cup

Muffin, small	1 (1½ oz)
Pancake, 4 inches across	2
Popcorn, microwave	3 cups
Sandwich crackers, cheese or peanut butter filling	3
Stuffing, bread (prepared)	⅓ cup
Taco shell, 6 inches across	2
Waffle, 4½ inches square	1
Whole-wheat crackers, fat added	4–6 (1 oz)

Starches often swell in cooking, so a small amount of uncooked starch will become a much larger amount of cooked food. The following table shows some of the changes.

Food (Starch Group)	Uncooked	Cooked
Oatmeal	3 Tbsp	½ cup
Cream of Wheat	2 Tbsp	½ cup
Grits	3 Tbsp	½ cup
Rice	2 Tbsp	½ cup
Spaghetti	¼ cup	½ cup
Noodles	⅓ cup	½ cup
Macaroni	¼ cup	½ cup
Dried beans	¼ cup	½ cup
Dried peas	¼ cup	½ cup
Lentils	3 Tbsp	½ cup

Common Measurements

3 tsp = 1 Tbsp
4 Tbsp = ¼ cup
5⅓ Tbsp = ⅓ cup
4 ounces = ½ cup
8 ounces = 1 cup
1 cup = ½ pint

ONE FRUIT EXCHANGE EQUALS

**15 grams carbohydrate and
60 calories.
The weight includes skin, core,
seeds, and rind**

FRUIT

SERVING SIZE

Apple, unpeeled, small	1 (4 oz)
Applesauce, unsweetened	½ cup
Apples, dried	4 rings

FRUIT	SERVING SIZE
Apricots, fresh	4 whole (5½ oz)
Apricots, dried	8 halves
Apricots, canned	½ cup
Banana, extra small	1 (4 oz)
Blackberries	¾ cup
Blueberries	¾ cup
Cantaloupe, small melon	⅓ melon (11 oz) or 1 cup cubed
Cherries, sweet, fresh	12 (3 oz)
Cherries, sweet, canned	½ cup
Dates	3
Dried fruits (blueberries, cherries, cranberries, mixed fruit, raisins)	2 Tbsp
Figs, fresh	1½ large or 2 medium (3½ oz)
Figs, dried	1½
Fruit cocktail	½ cup
Grapefruit, large	½ (11 oz)
Grapefruit sections, canned	¾ cup
Grapes, small	17 (3 oz)
Honeydew melon	1 slice (10 oz) or 1 cup cubed
Kiwi	1 (3½ oz)
Mandarin oranges, canned	¾ cup
Mango, small	½ fruit (5½ oz) or ½ cup
Nectarine, small	1 (5 oz)
Orange, small	1 (6½ oz)
Papaya	½ fruit (8 oz) or 1 cup cubed
Peach, medium, fresh	1 (6 oz)
Peaches, canned	½ cup
Pear, large, fresh	½ (4 oz)
Pears, canned	½ cup
Pineapple, fresh	¾ cup
Pineapple, canned	½ cup
Plums, small	2 (5 oz)
Plums, canned	½ cup
Prunes, dried	3
Raisins	2 Tbsp
Raspberries	1 cup
Strawberries	1¼ cup whole berries
Tangerines, small	2 (8 oz)
Watermelon	1 slice (13½ oz) or 1¼ cup cubes

FRUIT JUICE

	SERVING SIZE
Apple juice/cider	½ cup
Cranberry juice cocktail	⅓ cup
Cranberry juice cocktail, reduced-calorie	1 cup
Fruit juice blends, 100% juice	⅓ cup
Grape juice	⅓ cup
Grapefruit juice	½ cup
Orange juice	½ cup
Pineapple juice	½ cup
Prune juice	⅓ cup

ONE MILK EXCHANGE EQUALS

12 grams carbohydrate and 8 grams protein.

FAT-FREE AND LOW-FAT MILK
(0–3 grams fat per serving)

	SERVING SIZE
Fat-free milk	1 cup
½% milk	1 cup
1% milk	1 cup
Fat-free or low-fat buttermilk	1 cup
Lactaid, acidophilus milk	1 cup
Evaporated fat-free milk	½ cup
Fat-free dry milk	⅓ cup dry
Plain nonfat yogurt	⅔ cup (6 oz)
Nonfat or low-fat fruit-flavored yogurt sweetened with aspartame or with a non-nutritive sweetener	⅔ cup (6 oz)

REDUCED-FAT
(5 grams fat per serving)

	SERVING SIZE
2% milk	1 cup
Plain low-fat yogurt	⅔ cup (6 oz)
Sweet acidophilus milk	1 cup
Kefir	1 cup
Lactaid	1 cup

WHOLE MILK
(8 grams fat per serving)

	SERVING SIZE
Whole milk	1 cup
Evaporated whole milk	½ cup
Goat's milk	1 cup
Kefir	1 cup
Yogurt, plain	8 oz

DAIRY-LIKE FOODS

Chocolate milk, fat-free	1 cup
Chocolate milk, whole	1 cup
Eggnog, whole milk	½ cup
Rice drink, flavored, low-fat or plain, fat-free	1 cup
Smoothies, flavored, regular	10 oz
Soy milk, light	1 cup
Soy milk, regular, plain	1 cup
Yogurt, and juice blends	1 cup
Yogurt, low carbohydrate (less than 6 grams carbohydrate per choice)	⅔ cup (6 oz)
Yogurt, with fruit, low-fat	⅔ cup (6 oz)

ONE EXCHANGE EQUALS

15 grams carbohydrate, or 1 starch, or 1 fruit, or 1 milk.

Food	Serving Size	Exchanges Per Serving
Angel food cake, unfrosted	$\frac{1}{12}$ th cake	2 carbohydrates
Brownie, small, unfrosted	1¼ in. square	1 carbohydrate, 1 fat
Cake, unfrosted	2 in. square (1 oz.)	1 carbohydrate, 1 fat
Cake, frosted	2 in. square (2 oz.)	2 carbohydrates, 1 fat
Cookie, fat-free	2 small	1 carbohydrate
Cookie or sandwich cookie with creme filling	2 small	1 carbohydrate, 1 fat
Cranberry sauce, jellied	¼ cup	1½ carbohydrates
Cupcake, frosted	1 small	2 carbohydrates, 1 fat
Doughnut, plain cake	1 medium (1½ oz)	1½ carbohydrates, 2 fats
Doughnut, glazed	3¾ in. across (2 oz)	2 carbohydrates, 2 fats
Fruit juice bars, frozen, 100% juice	1 bar (3 oz)	1 carbohydrate
Fruit snacks, chewy (puréed fruit concentrate)	1 roll (¾ oz)	1 carbohydrate
Fruit spreads, 100% fruit	1 Tbsp	1 carbohydrate
Gelatin, regular	½ cup	1 carbohydrate
Gingersnaps	3	1 carbohydrate
Granola bar	1 bar	1 carbohydrate, 1 fat
Granola bar, fat-free	1 bar	2 carbohydrates

ONE EXCHANGE EQUALS

15 grams carbohydrate,
or 1 starch, or 1 fruit,
or 1 milk.

Food	Serving Size	Exchanges Per Serving
Honey	1 Tbsp	1 carbohydrate
Hummus	⅓ cup	1 carbohydrate, 1 fat
Ice cream	½ cup	1 carbohydrate, 2 fats
Ice cream, light	½ cup	1 carbohydrate, 1 fat
Ice cream, fat-free, no sugar added	½ cup	1 carbohydrate
Jam or jelly, regular	1 Tbsp	1 carbohydrate
Milk, chocolate, whole	1 cup	2 carbohydrates, 1 fat
Pie, fruit, 2 crusts	⅙ pie	3 carbohydrates, 2 fats
Pie, pumpkin or custard	⅛ pie (8-inch pie)	1½ carbohydrates, 1½ fats
Potato chips	12–18 (1 oz)	1 carbohydrate, 2 fats
Pudding, regular (made with low-fat milk)	½ cup	2 carbohydrates
Pudding, sugar-free (made with low-fat milk)	½ cup	1 carbohydrate
Salad dressing, fat-free*	¼ cup	1 carbohydrate
Sherbet, sorbet	½ cup	2 carbohydrates
Spaghetti or pasta sauce, canned*	½ cup	1 carbohydrate, 1 fat
Sugar	1 Tbsp	1 carbohydrate
Sweet roll or Danish	1 (2½ oz)	2½ carbohydrates, 2 fats
Syrup, light	2 Tbsp	1 carbohydrate
Syrup, regular	1 Tbsp	1 carbohydrate
Syrup, regular	¼ cup	4 carbohydrates
Tortilla chips	6–12 (1 oz)	1 carbohydrate, 2 fats
Vanilla wafers	5 cookies	1 carbohydrate, 1 fat
Yogurt, frozen, low-fat, fat-free	⅓ cup	1 carbohydrate, 0–1 fat
Yogurt, frozen, fat-free, no sugar added	½ cup	1 carbohydrate
Yogurt, low-fat with fruit	1 cup	3 carbohydrates, 0–1 fat

*= 400 mg or more of sodium per exchange

ONE VEGETABLE EXCHANGE EQUALS

5 grams carbohydrate,
2 grams protein,
0 grams fat, and
25 calories.

NONSTARCHY VEGETABLES

(½ cup cooked or 1 cup raw = 1 vegetable serving of all of the vegetables listed)

Artichoke
Artichoke hearts
Asparagus
Beans (green, wax, Italian)
Bean sprouts
Beets
Borscht
Broccoli
Brussels sprouts
Cabbage (green, bok choy, Chinese)
Carrots
Cauliflower
Celery
Chayote
Coleslaw, packaged, no dressing
Cucumber
Eggplant
Gourds (bitter, bottle, luffa, bitter melon)
Green onions or scallions
Greens (collard, kale, mustard, turnip)
Hearts of palm
Jicama
Kohlrabi
Leeks
Mixed vegetables (without corn, peas, or pasta)
Mung bean sprouts
Mushrooms, all kinds, fresh
Okra
Onions
Pea pods
Peppers (all varieties)
Radishes
Rutabaga
Salad greens (endive, escarole, lettuce, romaine, spinach)
Sauerkraut*
Soybean sprouts
Spinach

Squash (summer, crookneck, zucchini)
Sugar pea snaps
Swiss chard
Tomato
Tomatoes, canned
Tomato sauce*
Tomato/vegetable juice*
Turnips
Water chestnuts
Watercress
Yard-long beans

*= 400 mg or more sodium per exchange.

ONE EXCHANGE EQUALS

0 grams carbohydrate,
7 grams protein,
0–1 gram fat, and
35 calories.

VERY LEAN MEAT AND SUBSTITUTES LIST

(One very lean meat exchange is equal to any one of the following items.)

SERVING SIZE

Poultry: Chicken or turkey (white meat, no skin), Cornish hen (no skin)	1 oz
Fish: Fresh or frozen cod, flounder, haddock, halibut, trout; tuna fresh or canned in water	1 oz
Shellfish: Clams, crab, lobster, scallops, shrimp, imitation shellfish	1 oz
Game: Duck or pheasant (no skin), venison, buffalo, ostrich	1 oz
Cheese with 1 gram or less fat per ounce:	
Nonfat or low-fat cottage cheese	¼ cup
Fat-free cheese	1 oz
Other: Processed sandwich meats with 1 gram or less fat per ounce, such as deli thin-sliced meats, turkey ham, turkey kielbasa, turkey pastrami, shaved meats, chipped beef*	1 oz
Egg whites	2
Egg substitutes, plain	¼ cup
Hot dogs with 1 gram or less fat per ounce*	1 oz
Kidney (high in cholesterol)	1 oz
Sausage with 3 grams of fat or less per ounce	1 oz

(Count as one very lean meat and one starch exchange.)

Beans, peas, lentils (cooked)	½ cup

*= 400 mg or more sodium per exchange

0 grams carbohydrate,
7 grams protein,
3 grams fat, and
55 calories.

LEAN MEAT AND SUBSTITUTES LIST

(One lean meat exchange is equal to any one of the following items.)

SERVING SIZE

Beef: USDA Select or Choice grades of lean beef trimmed of fat, such as round, sirloin, and flank steak; tenderloin; roast (rib, chuck, rump); steak (T-bone, porterhouse, cubed), ground round	1 oz
Pork: Lean pork, such as fresh ham; canned, cured, or boiled ham; Canadian bacon*; tenderloin, center loin chop	1 oz
Lamb: Roast, chop, leg	1 oz
Veal: Lean chop, roast	1 oz
Poultry: Chicken, turkey (dark meat, no skin), chicken (white meat, with skin), domestic duck or goose (well drained of fat, no skin)	1 oz
Fish: Herring (uncreamed or smoked)	1 oz
Oysters, fresh or frozen	6 medium
Salmon (fresh or canned), catfish	1 oz
Sardines (canned)	2 medium
Tuna (canned in oil, drained)	1 oz
Game: Goose (no skin), rabbit	1 oz
Cheese: 4.5%-fat cottage cheese	¼ cup
Grated Parmesan	2 Tbsp
Cheeses with 3 grams or less fat per ounce	1 oz
Other: Hot dogs with 3 grams or less fat per ounce*	1 oz
Processed sandwich meat with 3 grams or less fat per ounce, such as turkey pastrami or kielbasa	1 oz
Liver, heart (high in cholesterol)	1 oz

ONE EXCHANGE EQUALS

0 grams carbohydrate,
7 grams protein,
5 grams fat, and
75 calories.

MEDIUM-FAT MEAT AND SUBSTITUTES LIST

(One medium-fat meat exchange is equal to any one of the following items.)

SERVING SIZE

Beef: Most beef products fall into this category (ground beef, meatloaf, corned beef, short ribs, prime grades of meat trimmed of fat such as prime rib, tongue)	1 oz
Pork: Top loin, chop, Boston butt, cutlet	1 oz
Lamb: Rib roast, ground	1 oz
Veal: Cutlet (ground or cubed, no breading)	1 oz
Poultry: Chicken (dark meat, with skin), ground turkey or ground chicken, fried chicken (with skin), dove, pheasant, wild duck, or goose	1 oz
Fish: Any fried fish product	1 oz
Cheese: With 5 grams or less fat per ounce, reduced fat cheeses, pasteurized processed cheese spread	
Feta	1 oz
Mozzarella	1 oz
Ricotta	¼ cup (2 oz)
Other:	
Egg (high in cholesterol, limit to 3 per week)	1
Sausage with 5 grams or less fat per ounce	1 oz
Soy Milk	1 cup
Tempeh	¼ cup
Tofu	4 oz or ½ cup

*= 400 mg or more sodium per exchange

ONE EXCHANGE EQUALS

0 grams carbohydrate,
7 grams protein,
8 grams fat, and
100 calories.

HIGH-FAT MEAT AND SUBSTITUTES LIST

(One high-fat meat exchange is equal to any one of the following items.)

Remember these items are high in saturated fat, cholesterol, and calories and may raise blood cholesterol levels if eaten on a regular basis.

Pork: Spareribs, ground pork, pork sausage	1 oz
Cheese: All regular cheeses, such as American*, cheddar, Monterey Jack, Swiss	1 oz
Other: Processed sandwich meats with 8 grams or less fat per ounce, such as bologna, pimento loaf, salami	1 oz
Sausage, such as bratwurst, Italian, knockwurst, Polish, smoked	1 oz
Hot dog (turkey or chicken)*	1 (10/lb)
Bacon	3 slices (20 slices/lb)

(Count as one high-fat meat plus one fat exchange.

Hot dog (beef, pork, or combination)*	1 (10/lb)

Count as one high-fat meat plus two fat exchanges.

Peanut butter (contains unsaturated fat)	2 Tbsp

ONE FAT EXCHANGE EQUALS

5 grams fat and 45 calories.

MONOUNSATURATED FATS LIST

Avocado, medium	⅛ (1 oz)
Oil (canola, olive, peanut)	1 tsp
Olives: ripe (black)	8 large
green, stuffed*	10 large
Nuts:	
almonds, cashews	6 nuts
Brazil	2 nuts
filberts (hazelnuts	5 nuts
mixed (50% peanuts)	6 nuts
peanuts	10 nuts
pecans	4 halves
pistachios	16 nuts
Peanut butter, smooth or crunchy	1½ tsp
Sesame seeds	1 Tbsp
Tahini paste	2 tsp

* = 400 mg or more sodium per exchange

ONE FAT EXCHANGE EQUALS

5 grams fat, and
45 calories.

POLYUNSATURATED FATS LIST	SERVING SIZE
Margarine: stick, tub, or squeeze	1 tsp
lower-fat (30% to 50% vegetable oil, trans fat-free)	1 Tbsp
Mayonnaise: regular	1 tsp
reduced-fat	1 Tbsp
Mayonnaise-style salad dressing, reduced-fat	1 Tbsp
Mayonnaise-style salad dressing, regular	2 tsp
Nuts, walnuts, English	4 halves
Oil (corn, cottonseed, flaxseed, grape seed, safflower, soybean,sunflower)	1 tsp
Salad dressing: regular*	1 Tbsp
reduced-fat	2 Tbsp
Miracle Whip Salad Dressing®: regular	2 tsp
reduced-fat	1 Tbsp
Seeds: pumpkin, sunflower, sesame seeds	1 Tbsp
Tahini or sesame paste	2 tsps

*= 400 mg or more sodium per exchange

ONE FAT EXCHANGE EQUALS

5 grams fat, and
45 calories.

SATURATED FATS LIST**	SERVING SIZE
Bacon, cooked, regular or turkey	1 slice (20 slices/lb)
Bacon, grease	1 tsp
Butter: stick	1 tsp
whipped	2 tsp
reduced-fat	1 Tbsp
Chitterlings, boiled	2 Tbsp (½ oz)
Coconut milk, light	⅓ cup
Regular	1½ Tbsp
Coconut, sweetened, shredded	2 Tbsp
Cream, half and half	2 Tbsp
Heavy	1 Tbsp
Light	1½ Tbsp
Whipped	2 Tbsp
Whipped, pressurized	¼ cup
Cream cheese: regular	1 Tbsp (½ oz)
reduced-fat	2 Tbsp (1 oz)
Fatback or salt pork, see below†	

Shortening or lard	1 tsp
Sour cream: regular	2 Tbsp
reduced-fat or light	3 Tbsp

**Saturated fats can raise blood cholesterol levels

†Use a piece 1 in. x 1 in. x ¼ in. if you plan to eat the fatback cooked with vegetables. Use a piece 2 in. x 1 in. x ½ in. when eating only the vegetables with the fatback removed.

Free Foods List

A *free food* is any food or drink that contains less than 20 calories or less than 5 grams of carbohydrate per serving. Foods with a serving size listed should be limited to three servings per day. Be sure to spread them out throughout the day. If you eat all three servings at one time, it could affect your blood glucose level. Foods listed without a serving size can be eaten as often as you like.

FAT-FREE OR REDUCED-FAT FOODS	SERVING SIZE
Cream cheese, fat-free	1 Tbsp (½ oz)
Creamers, nondairy, liquid	1 Tbsp
Creamers, nondairy, powdered	2 tsp
Margarine, fat-free	4 Tbsp
Margarine, reduced-fat	1 tsp
Mayonnaise, fat-free	1 Tbsp
Mayonnaise, reduced-fat	1 tsp
Miracle Whip®, nonfat	1 Tbsp
Miracle Whip®, reduced-fat	1 tsp
Nonstick cooking spray	
Salad dressing, fat-free	1 Tbsp
Salad dressing, fat-free, Italian	2 Tbsp
Salsa	¼ cup
Sour cream, fat-free, reduced-fat	1 Tbsp
Whipped topping, regular or light	2 Tbsp

SUGAR-FREE OR LOW-SUGAR FOODS	SERVING SIZE
Candy, hard, sugar-free	1 candy
Gelatin dessert, sugar-free	
Gelatin, unflavored	
Gum, sugar-free	
Jam or jelly, low-sugar or light	2 tsp
Rhubarb, sweetened with sugar substitute	½ cup
Salad greens	
Sugar substitutes†Syrup, sugar-free	2 Tbsp

†See Artificial Sweeteners, next page.

ARTIFICIAL SWEETENERS

Sugar substitutes, alternatives, or replacements that are approved by the Food and Drug Administration (FDA) are safe to use. Common brand names include:
Equal® and Nutrasweet® (aspartame)
Splenda (sucralose)
Sugar Twin®, Sweet-10®, Sweet 'n Low®, and Sprinkle Sweet® (saccharin)
Sweet One® (acesulfame-K)

Although each sweetener is tested for safety before it can be marketed and sold, use a variety of sweeteners and in moderate amounts.

DRINKS

Bouillon, broth, consommé*
Bouillon or broth, low-sodium
Carbonated or mineral water
Club soda
Cocoa powder, unsweetened   1 Tbsp
Coffee, unsweetened or with sugar substitute
Diet soft drinks, sugar-free
Drink mixes, sugar-free
Tea, unsweetened or with sugar substitute
Tonic water, sugar-free
Water, flavored, carbohydrate free

CONDIMENTS

Catsup	1 Tbsp
Horseradish	
Lemon juice	
Lime juice	
Mustard	
Pickles, dill*	1½ large
sweet, bread and butter	2 slices
sweet, gherkin	¾ oz
Salsa	¼ cup
Soy sauce, regular or light*	1 Tbsp
Sweet and sour sauce	2 tsp
Taco sauce	1 Tbsp
Vinegar	
Yogurt, any type	2 Tbsp

* = 400 mg or more of sodium per exchange

SEASONINGS

Be careful with seasonings that contain sodium or are salts, such as garlic or celery salt, and lemon pepper.

Flavoring extracts
Garlic
Herbs, fresh or dried
Nonstick cooking spray
Pimento
Spices
Tabasco® or hot pepper sauce
Wine, used in cooking
Worcestershire sauce

FREE SNACKS

These foods in these serving sizes are perfect free-food snacks.

5 baby carrots and celery sticks
¼ cup blueberries
½ oz sliced cheese, fat-free
10 goldfish-style crackers
2 saltine-type crackers
1 frozen cream pop, sugar-free
½ oz lean meat
1 cup light popcorn
1 vanilla wafer

Combination Foods

Many of the foods we eat are mixed together in various combinations. These combination foods do not fit into any one exchange list. Often it is hard to tell what is in a casserole dish or prepared food item. This is a list of exchanges for some typical combination foods. This list will help you fit these foods into your meal plan. Ask your dietitian for information about any other combination foods you would like to eat.

ENTREES

Food	Serving Size	Count as
Tuna noodle casserole, lasagna, spaghetti with meatballs, chili with beans, macaroni and cheese*	1 cup (8 oz)	2 carbohydrates + 2 medium-fat meats
Chow mein (without noodles or rice)*	2 cups (16 oz)	1 carbohydrate + 2 lean meats

Pizza, cheese, thin crust*	¼ of 10 in. (5 oz)	2 carbohydrates, 2 medium-fat meats, 1 fat
Pizza, meat topping, thin crust*	¼ of 10 in. (5 oz)	2 carbohydrates + 2 medium-fat meats, 2 fats
Pot pie	1 (7 oz)	2 carbohydrates +1 medium-fat meat + 4 fats

FROZEN MEALS/ENTREES

Food	Serving Size	Count as
Salisbury steak with gravy, mashed potato*	1 (11 oz)	2 carbohydrates + 3 medium-fat meats + 3–4 fats
Turkey with gravy, mashed potato, dressing*	1 (11 oz)	2 carbohydrates + 2 medium-fat meats + 2 fats
Entree with less than 300 calories*	1 (8 oz)	2 carbohydrates + 3 lean meats

SOUPS

Food	Serving Size	Count as
Bean*	1 cup	1 carbohydrate + 1 very lean meat
Chowder(made with water)*	1 cup	1 carbohydrate + 1 lean meat + 1½ fats
Cream (made with water)*	1 cup (8 oz)	1 carbohydrate + 1 fat
Miso soup*	1 cup	½ carbohydrate + 1 fat
Split pea (made with water)*	½ cup (4 oz)	1 carbohydrate
Tomato (made with water)*	1 cup (8 oz)	1 carbohydrate
Vegetable beef, chicken noodle, or other broth-type*	1 cup (8 oz)	1 carbohydrate

*= 600 mg or more sodium per exchange

SALADS (DELI-STYLE)

Food	Serving Size	Count as
Coleslaw	½ cup	1 carbohydrate + 1½ fats
Macaroni/pasta salad	½ cup	2 carbohydrates + 3 fats
Potato salad	½ cup	1½ -2 carbohydrates + 1-2 fats

Fast Foods

BREAKFAST SANDWICHES

Food	Serving Size	Count as
Egg, cheese, meat, english muffin	1 sandwich	2 carbohydrates + 2 medium-fat meats
Sausage biscuit sandwich	1 sandwich	2 carbohydrates + 2 high-fat meats + 3½ fats

MAIN DISHES/ENTREES

Food	Serving Size	Count as
Burrito (beef and beans)	1 (about 8 oz)	3 carbohydrates + 3 medium-fat meats + 3 fats
Chicken breast, breaded and fried	1 (about 5 oz)	1 carbohydrate + 4 medium-fat meats
Chicken drumstick, breaded and fried	1 (about 2 oz)	2 medium-fat meats
Chicken nuggets	6 (about 3½ oz)	1 carbohydrate + 2 medium-fat meats + 1 fat
Chicken thigh, breaded and fried	1 (about 4 oz)	½ carbohydrate + 3 medium-fat meats + 1½ fats
Chicken wings, hot	6 (5 oz)	5 medium-fat meats + 1½ fats

ORIENTAL (ASIAN)

Food	Serving Size	Count as
Beef/chicken/shrimp with vegetables in sauce	1 cup (about 5 oz)	1 carbohydrate + 1 lean meat + 1 fat
Egg roll, meat	1 (about 3 oz)	1 carbohydrate + 1 lean meat + 1 fat
Fried rice, meatless	½ cup	1½ carbohydrates + 1½ fats
Meat and sweet sauce (orange chicken)	1 cup	3 carbohydrates + 3 medium-fat meats + 2 fats
Noodles and vegetables in sauce (chow mein, lo mein)	1 cup	2 carbohydrates + 1 fat

PIZZA

Food	Serving Size	Count as
cheese, pepperoni, regular crust	⅛ of a 14 inch (about 4 oz)	2 ½ carbohydrates + 1 medium-fat meat + 1½ fats
cheese/vegetarian, thin crust	¼ of a 12 inch (about 6 oz)	2 ½ carbohydrates + 2 medium-fat meats + ½ fat

SANDWICHES

Food	Serving Size	Count as
Chicken sandwich, grilled	1	3 carbohydrates + 4 lean meats
Chicken sandwich, crispy	1	3½ carbohydrates + 3 medium-fat meats + 1 fat
Fish sandwich with tartar sauce	1	2½ carbohydrates + 2 medium-fat meats + 2 fats
Hamburger: large with cheese	1	2½ carbohydrates + 4 medium-fat meats + 1 fat
regular	1	2 carbohydrates + 1 medium-fat meat + 1 fat
Hot dog with bun	1	1 carbohydrate + 1 high-fat meat + 1 fat
Submarine sandwich, less than 6 grams fat	6-inch sub	3 carbohydrates + 2 lean meats
regular	6-inch sub	3½ carbohydrates + 2 medium-fat meats + 1 fat
Taco, hard or soft shell (meat and cheese)	1 small	1 carbohydrate + 1 medium-fat meat + 1½ fats

SALADS

Food	Serving Size	Count as
Salad, main dish (grilled chicken type, no dressing or croutons)	Salad	1 carbohydrate + 4 lean meats
Salad, side, no dressing or cheese	Small (about 5 oz)	1 vegetable

SIDES/APPETIZERS

Food	Serving Size	Count as
French fries, restaurant style	small	3 carbohydrates + 3 fats
	medium	4 carbohydrates + 4 fats
	large	5 carbohydrates + 6 fats
Nachos with cheese	small (about 4½ oz)	2½ carbohydrates + 4 fats
Onion rings	1 serving (about 3 oz)	2½ carbohydrates + 3 fats

DESSERTS

Food	Serving Size	Count as
Milkshake, any flavor	12 oz	6 carbohydrates + 2 fats
Soft-serve ice cream cone	1 small	2½ carbohydrates + 1 fat

*See the Starch list and Sweets, Desserts, and Other Carbohydrates list for foods such as bagels and muffins

Alcohol

In general, 1 alcohol choice (½ oz absolute alcohol) has about 100 calories.

If you choose to drink alcohol, you should limit it to 1 drink or less per day for women, and 2 drinks or less per day for men. To reduce your risk of low blood glucose (hypoglycemia), especially if you take insulin or a diabetes pill that increases insulin, always drink alcohol with food. While alcohol, by itself does not directly affect blood glucose, be aware of the carbohydrate (for example, in mixed drinks, beer, and wine) that may raise your blood glucose. Check with your RD if you would like to fit alcohol into your meal plan.

Beverage	Serving Size	Count as
Beer		
light (4.2%)	12 fl oz	1 alcohol equivalent + ½ carbohydrate
regular (4.9%)	12 fl oz	1 alcohol equivalent + 1 carbohydrate
Distilled spirits: vodka, rum, gin, whiskey 80 or 86 proof	1½ fl oz	1 alcohol equivalent
Liqueur, coffee (53 proof)	1 fl oz	1 alcohol equivalent+ 1 carbohydrate
Sake	1 fl oz	½ alcohol equivalent
Wine		
dessert (sherry)	3½ fl oz	1 alcohol equivalent + 1 carbohydrate
dry, red, or white (10%)	5 fl oz	1 alcohol equivalent

PREPARED PRODUCTS

BREAD

	PRODUCT	AMOUNT	CALORIES	EXCHANGE
Best Foods, CPC International	Argo Cornstarch	2 T. (30 mL)	70	1 bread
	Duryea's Cornstarch	2 T. (30 mL)	70	1 bread
	Kingsford Cornstarch	2 T. (30 mL)	70	1 bread
	Presto Self-Rising Cake Flour	2½ T. (35 mL)	60	1 bread
Creamette Co.	Egg Noodles (cooked)	1 c. (250 mL)	220	3 bread
	Macaroni and Cheese Dinner (cooked)	1 c. (250 mL)	240	3 bread 2 fat
	Pasta Misc. (cooked)	1 c. (250 mL)	210	3 bread
General Foods	Stove Top Stuffing Mixes	½ c. (125 mL)	180	1½ bread 2 fat
General Mills	Bisquick	2 oz. (60 g)	70	2½ bread 1½ fat
	POTATOES: 1 portion, prepared as directed			
	Au Gratin		150	1½ bread 1 fat
	Creamed		160	1½ bread 1 fat
	Hash Browns with Onions		150	1½ bread 1 fat
	Julienne		130	1 bread 1 fat
	Potato Buds		130	1 bread 1 fat
	Scalloped		150	1½ bread 1 fat
	Sour Cream n' Chive		140	1 bread 1 fat

Pillsbury				
PIE CRUSTS: Prepared according to basic recipe				
	Mix or Stick	⅙ crust	145	1 bread 1 fat
OTHER BREADS: Prepared according to basic recipe				
	Hot Roll Mix	1 roll	95	1 bread ½ fat
	Hotloaf	1 slice	90	1 bread ½ fat
HUNGRY JACK BISCUITS				
	Butter Tastin'	1 biscuit	190	1½ bread 2 fat
	Flaky	2 biscuits	180	1½ bread 2 fat
	Flaky Buttermilk	2 biscuits	180	1½ bread 2 fat
	Fluffy Buttermilk	2 biscuits	190	1½ bread 2 fat
PILLSBURY BISCUITS				
	Buttermilk	2 biscuits	110	1½ bread
	Country Style	2 biscuits	110	1½ bread
	Flaky Tenderflake Buttermilk Dinner	2 biscuits	120	1 bread 2 fat
	Tenderflake Baking Powder Dinner	2 biscuits	120	1 bread 1 fat
HUNGRY JACK POTATOES: Prepared according to basic recipe				
	Mashed Potato Flakes	½ c. (125 mL)	140	1 bread 1½ fat
HUNGRY JACK PANCAKE & WAFFLE MIXES: 1 pancake, 4 in. (10 cm) prepared according to basic recipe				
	Blueberry		113	1 bread 1 fat
	Buttermilk		80	½ bread 1 fat
DINNER ROLLS				
	Oven Lovin'	2 rolls	110	1 bread ½ fat
	Pillsbury Crescent	2 rolls	190	1½ bread 2 fat
MUFFINS				
	Apple, Cinnamon, Bran, or Corn	1 muffin	120	1 bread 1 fat
WIENER WRAPS				
	Cheese	1 wrap	70	½ bread ½ fat
	Plain	1 wrap	60	½ bread ½ fat

MEAT

	PRODUCT	AMOUNT	CALORIES	EXCHANGE
Hormel	Coarse-Ground Bologna	2 oz.	150	2 high-fat meat
	Chopped Ham	1 oz.	70	1 lean meat ½ fat
	Deviled Ham	1 oz.	70	½ lean meat
	Kolbase Polish Sausage	3 oz.	70	2 high-fat meat 1 fat
	Meat or Beef Wieners	1	140	1 high-fat meat
	Spam	3 oz.	260	1½ medium-fat meat ½ vegetable
	Tender Chunk Chicken	3 oz.	110	2 lean meat
	Tender Chunk Ham	3 oz.	140	2 medium-fat meat
	Tender Chunk Turkey	3 oz. (90 g)	90	2 lean meat
Oscar Mayer	Beef Bologna	1 slice	75	½ meat 1 fat
	Beef Cotto Salami	1 slice	50	½ meat ½ fat
	Beef Franks	1 slice	140	½ meat 2 fat
	Braunschweiger	1	70	½ meat 1 fat
	Chopped Ham	1 slice	65	½ meat ½ fat
	Cooked Ham	1 slice	30	½ meat
	Hard Salami	1 slice	35	¼ meat ½ fat
	Honey Loaf	1 slice	35	½ meat
	Jubilee Canned Ham	1 oz.	35	½ meat
	Little Friers Pork Sausage	1	65	½ meat 1 fat
	New England Brand Sausage	1	35	½ meat
	Sandwich Spread	1 oz. (30 g)	60	½ fat

CASSEROLES AND ONE-DISH MEALS

	PRODUCT	AMOUNT	CALORIES	EXCHANGE
Franco-American	Beef Ravioli in Meat Sauce	7½ oz. (225 g)	220	1 vegetable 2 bread 1 lean meat
	Elbow Macaroni & Cheese	7¼ oz. (220 g)	180	2 bread 1 fat
	Rotini in Tomato Sauce	7½ oz. (225 g)	200	1 vegetable 1 fat
	Spaghetti in Meat Sauce	7¾ oz. (230 g)	220	1 vegetable 1 bread 1 lean meat 1 fat
	Spaghetti-O's in Tomato & Cheese Sauce	7½ oz. (225 g)	160	1 vegetable 1 bread 1 lean meat 1 fat
	HAMBURGER HELPER: 1 portion, prepared as directed			
General Mills	Beef Noodle		320	2 bread 2 medium-fat meat, ½ fat
	Cheeseburger Macaroni		360	1½ bread ½ milk 2 medium-fat meat, 1 fat
	Lasagne		330	2 bread 2 medium-fat meat, ½ fat
	Hamburger Pizza Dish		340	2 bread 2 medium-fat meat, ½ fat
	Hamburger Stew		290	1 bread 1 vegetable 2 medium-fat meat, 1 fat
	Potato Stroganoff		330	2 bread 2 medium-fat meat, ½ fat
	Rice Oriental	8-oz. pkg. (240-g pkg.)	340	2 bread 2 medium-fat meat, ½ fat
	Spaghetti		330	2 bread 2 medium-fat meat, ½ fat
	TUNA HELPER: 1 portion, prepared as directed			
	Country Dumplings 'n Tuna		230	2 bread 1 lean meat ½ fat
	Creamy Noodles 'n Tuna		280	2 bread 1 lean meat 1½ fat
	Noodles, Cheese Sauce 'n Tuna		230	1½ bread ½ milk 1 lean meat ½ fat

	CASEROLES AND SIDE DISHES: 1 portion, prepared as directed			
General Mills	Macaroni & Cheese		310	2 bread ½ milk 3 fat
	Noodles Romanoff		230	1 bread ½ milk 2½ fat
	Noodles Stroganoff		230	1½ bread ½ milk 2 fat
	SHORT ORDERS: 7½-oz. (225-g) can			
Hormel	Beans 'n Wieners		290	1 high-fat meat 1 fat 2 bread
	Beef Goulash		230	2 medium-fat meat 1 bread
	Chili with Beans		300	2 high-fat meat 1½ bread
	Lasagne		260	1 high-fat meat 1½ fat 1½ bread
	Spaghetti 'n Beef		240	1 high-fat meat 1 fat 1½ bread
	FROZEN MEAT PIES: 1 complete pie			
Swanson	Beef	8 oz. (240 g)	430	3 bread 1 lean meat 4 fat
	Chicken and Turkey	8 oz. (240 g)	450	3 bread 1 lean meat 4 fat
	Macaroni and Cheese	7 oz. (210 g)	230	2 bread 1 lean meat 1 fat
	HUNGRY MAN MEAT PIES: 1 complete pie			
	Beef	16 oz. (480 g)	770	1 vegetable 4 bread 3 lean meat 7 fat
	Chicken	16 oz. (480 g)	780	1 vegetable 4 bread 3 lean meat 7 fat
	Turkey	16 oz. (480 g)	790	1 vegetable 4 bread 3 lean meat 7 fat

	ENTREES: 1 complete entrée			
Swanson	Chicken Nibbles with French Fries	6 oz. (180 g)	370	2 bread 2 lean meat 3 fat
	Fried Chicken with Whipped Potatoes	7 oz. (210 g)	360	2 bread 2 lean meat 2 fat
	Gravy & Sliced Beef with Whipped Potatoes	8 oz. (240 g)	190	1½ bread 1 lean meat 1 fat
	Spaghetti with Breaded Veal	8¼ oz. (250 g)	290	2 bread 1 lean meat 3 fat
	Turkey/Gravy/Dressing with Whipped Potatoes	8¾ oz. (280 g)	260	2 bread 2 lean meat
	HUNGRY MAN ENTREES			
	Barbecue Chicken with Whipped Potato	12 oz. (360 g)	550	3 bread 4 lean meat 3 fat
	Sliced Beef with Whipped Potatoes	12¼ oz. (370 g)	330	1½ bread 4 lean meat
	Turkey/Gravy/Dressing with Whipped Potatoes	13¼ oz. (400 g)	380	2 bread 4 lean meat

SANDWICHES AND SNACKS

	PRODUCT	AMOUNT	CALORIES	EXCHANGE
Best Foods, CPC International	Skippy Dry-Roasted Peanuts, Cashews, Mixed Nuts	1 oz. (30 g)	165	1 medium-fat meat 2 fat
General Mills	Beef Jerky	1 strip	25	½ lean meat
Kraft Pizza	Cheese	¼ pizza	250	2½ bread 1 fat 1 medium-fat meat
	Sausage	¼ pizza	280	2½ bread 1 fat 1 medium-fat meat

Ore-Ida Foods	Onion Ringers	2 oz. (60 g)	160	1 bread 2 fat
	La Pizzeria Pizza, Pepperoni	5.3 oz. (160 g)	330	3 bread 1 fat 2 medium-fat meat
	La Pizzeria Pizza, Thick Crust, Cheese	6.2 oz (180 g)	410	3 bread 1 fat 2 medium-fat meat
Planters	OIL-ROASTED NUTS			
	Cashews	1 oz. (30 g)	180	1 bread 1 high-fat meat
	Mixed (with peanuts)	1 oz. (30 g)	185	1 fruit or ½ bread 1 high-fat meat
	Mixed (without peanuts)	1 oz. (30 g)	185	1 fruit or ½ bread 1 high-fat meat
	Peanuts	¾ oz. (22 g)	130	1 high-fat meat
	DRY ROASTED NUTS			
	Almonds	1 oz. (30 g)	185	1 fruit or ½ bread 1 high-fat meat
	Cashews	1 oz. (30 g)	180	1 fruit or ½ bread 1 high-fat meat
	Mixed	1 oz. (30 g)	175	1 fruit or ½ bread 1 high-fat meat
	Peanuts	1 oz. (30 g)	170	1 fruit or ½ bread 1 high-fat meat

FAST-FOOD ITEMS

	PRODUCT	AMOUNT	CALORIES	EXCHANGE
Burger King	Hamburger	1	240	2 bread 2 medium-fat meat 2 fat
	Double-Meat Hamburger	1	370	2 bread 3 medium-fat meat 3 fat
	Cheeseburger	1	310	2 bread 2 medium-fat meat 2 fat
	Double Meat Cheeseburger	1	420	2 bread 3 medium-fat meat 3 fat
	Whopper, Jr.	1	300	2 bread 2 medium-fat meat 2 fat
	Whopper, Jr. with Cheese	1	350	2 bread 2 medium-fat meat 3 fat
	Double Meat Whopper, Jr.	1	410	3 bread 4 lean meat 3 fat
	Double Meat Whopper, Jr. With Cheese	1	460	2 bread 3 medium-fat meat 3 fat
	Whopper	1	650	3½ bread 3 medium-fat meat 4½ fat
	Whopper with Cheese	1	760	3½ bread 3 medium-fat meat 5½ fat
	French Fries (small)	1	200	2 bread 2 fat
	French Fries (large)	1	320	3 bread 3 fat
	Onion Rings (small)	1	150	1 bread 1 vegetable 1½ fat
	Onion Rings (large)	1	220	2 bread 1 vegetable 2 fat

FAST-FOOD ITEMS

	FRIED CHICKEN, MASHED POTATO, COLESLAW, ROLLS		
Kentucky Fried Chicken	Original 3-piece dinner	830	4 bread 6 meat 2½ fat
	Crispy 3-piece dinner	1070	5 bread 6 meat 6½ fat
	Original 2-piece dinner	595	3½ bread 2 meat 1½ fat
	Crispy 2-piece dinner	665	3 bread 4½ meat 3½ fat

McDonalds	Hamburger	1	260	2 bread 1 medium-fat meat 1 fat
	Double Hamburger	1	350	2 bread 2 meat 1 fat
	Quarter Pounder	1	420	2½ bread 3 meat 1 fat
	Big Mac	1	550	3 bread 2 meat 4 fat
	French Fries	1	180	1½ bread 2 fat
	Chocolate Milk Shake	1	315	3½ bread 1½ fat

	CHEESE PIZZA			
Pizza Hut	Thick Crust, individual	1	1030	9½ bread 7½ meat
	Thin Crust, individual	1	1005	8½ bread 6 meat
	Thick Crust, 13 in.	half (32.5 cm)	900	7½ bread 7 meat
	Thin Crust, 13 in.	half (32.5 cm)	850	7 bread 5 meat

SAUCES AND SALAD DRESSINGS

	PRODUCT	AMOUNT	CALORIES	EXCHANGE
Best Foods, CPC International	Hellman's French	1 T. (15mL)	60	1 fat
	Hellman's Real Mayonnaise	1 t. (15 mL)	35	1 fat
	Hellman's Sandwich Spread	2 t. (10 mL)	40	1 fat
	Hellman's Spin Blend	1 t. (10 mL)	40	1 fat
	Hellman's Tartar Sauce	2 t. (15 mL)	50	1 fat
Campbell's	Beef Gravy	2 oz. (60 g)	30	1 fat
	Brown Gravy with Onions	2 oz. (60 g)	25	1 fat
	Chicken Gravy	2 oz. (60 g)	50	1 fat
	Chicken Giblet Gravy	2 oz. (60 g)	35	1 fat
	Mushroom Gravy	2 oz. (60 g)	35	1 fat
Chiffon Products	Lo-Cal French	1 T. (15 mL)	25	½ fat
	Lo-Cal Italian	1 T. (15 mL)	40	1 fat
	Seven Seas Salad Dressing	1 T. (15 mL)	70	1½ fat
Kraft Products	Miracle Whip	1 T. (15 mL)	70	1½ fat
	Real Mayonnaise	1 T. (15 mL)	10	2 fat
Pillsbury	Brown or Homestyle Gravy	½ c. (125 mL)	30	½ bread
	Chicken Gravy	½ c. (125 mL)	30	½ bread

INDEX

31901050615873